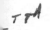

Receptors and
Recognition

Series B Volume 9

Neurotransmitter Receptors

Part 1
Amino Acids, Peptides
and Benzodiazepines

Edited by
S. J. Enna

Associate Professor of Pharmacology and Neurobiology
University of Texas Medical School at Houston

and

H. I. Yamamura

Professor of Pharmacology
University of Arizona
Health Sciences Center, Tucson,
Arizona

1980
LONDON AND NEW YORK
CHAPMAN AND HALL
150th Anniversary

First published 1980
by Chapman and Hall Ltd.,
11 New Fetter Lane, London EC4P 4EE

Published in the U.S.A. by
Chapman and Hall
in association with Methuen, Inc.,
733 Third Avenue, New York 10017

© *1980 Chapman and Hall*

Typeset by Preface Ltd., Salisbury
and printed in Great Britain
at the University Printing House, Cambridge

ISBN 0 412 16250 4

British Library Cataloguing in Publication Data
Receptors and recognition.
Series B, Vol. 9: Neurotransmitter
receptors. Part 1
1. Cell interaction
I. Cuatrecasas, Pedro
II. Greaves, Melvyn Francis
III. Enna, S J   IV. Yamamura, H I
V. Neurotransmitter receptors
574.8'76   QH604.2   80-40893

ISBN 0-412-16250-4

Receptors and Recognition

General Editors: P. Cuatrecasas and M.F. Greaves

About the series

Cellular Recognition – the process by which cells interact with, and respond to, molecular signals in their environment – plays a crucial role in virtually all important biological functions. These encompass fertilization, infectious interactions, embryonic development, the activity of the nervous system, the regulation of growth and metabolism by hormones and the immune response to foreign antigens. Although our knowledge of these systems has grown rapidly in recent years, it is clear that a full understanding of cellular recognition phenomena will require an integrated and multidisciplinary approach.

This series aims to expedite such an understanding by bringing together accounts by leading researchers of all biochemical, cellular and evolutionary aspects of recognition systems. This series will contain volumes of two types. First, there will be volumes containing about five reviews from different areas of the general subject written at a level suitable for all biologically oriented scientists (Receptors and Recognition, series A). Secondly, there will be more specialized volumes (Receptors and Recognition, series B), each of which will be devoted to just one particularly important area.

Receptors and Recognition

Series A

Published

Contents

Contributors

D.R. Burt, Department of Pharmacology, School of Medicine, The University of Maryland, Baltimore, Maryland, U.S.A.

S.R. Childers, Department of Pharmacology and Psychiatry, School of Medicine, The Johns Hopkins University, Baltimore, Maryland, U.S.A.

J.T. Coyle, Department of Pharmacology and Psychiatry, School of Medicine, The Johns Hopkins University, Baltimore, Maryland, U.S.A.

J.F. DeFrance, Departments of Pharmacology, Anatomy and Neurobiology, School of Medicine, The University of Texas at Houston, Houston, Texas, U.S.A.

S.J. Enna Departments of Pharmacology, Anatomy and Neurobiology, School of Medicine, The University of Texas at Houston, Houston, Texas, U.S.A.

M.R. Hanley, Department of Pharmacology, MRC.Neurochemistry Pharmacology Unit, University of Cambridge Medical School, Cambridge, U.K.

L.L. Iversen, Department of Pharmacology, MRC Neurochemistry Pharmacology Unit, University of Cambridge Medical School, Cambridge, U.K.

Contents of *Neurotransmitter Receptors Part 2*
Biogenic Amines

Preface

Since the discovery that neuronal transmission can be chemically mediated, a large number of compounds have been found in the mammalian central nervous system which appear to function as neurotransmitter agents. Recently, electrophysiological and biochemical methods have been developed which have enabled neuroscientists to classify better the myriad of neurotransmitter receptor sites in brain and to study their properties in finer detail. As a result of these investigations, a significant number of new discoveries have been made about the mechanisms involved in neurotransmitter receptor interactions, the role neurotransmitters play in the actions of pharmacological agents and in the pathogenesis of various neuropsychiatric disorders.

The present two volume text was compiled to summarize the information relating to the physiological, biochemical, pharmacological and functional characteristics of neurotransmitter receptor sites. While emphasis is placed on neurotransmitter receptors in the mammalian central nervous system, the characteristics of these receptors in other species, both vertebrate and invertebrate, are also discussed where appropriate. While these books cover the major classes of putative neurotransmitters – amino acids, peptides and biogenic amines – and are therefore broad in scope, each is discussed in a concise fashion to highlight the major points of historical and contemporary interest. In addition to outlining data, each chapter addresses current theories relating to the various aspects of receptor properties and function in an attempt to reveal the directions of future research and as a stimulus for other workers in the field. This work can serve not only as an introductory text for young neuroscientists, but should also be a valuable resource for more senior investigators as both a reference and research guide.

May, 1980

H.I. Yamamura
S.J. Enna

Neurotransmitter Receptors

Part 1
Amino Acids, Peptides
and Benzodiazepines

1 Excitatory Amino Acid Receptors

JOSEPH T. COYLE

Acknowledgements

The author is the recipient of RSDA Type II (KO3-MH00125) and receives research support from the USPHS grants MH-26654 and NS-13584 and the National Foundation March of Dimes. Helpful discussions with H. Shinozkai are gratefully acknowledged as well as the excellent secretarial assistance of Carol Kenyon.

Neurotransmitter Receptors Part 1
(*Receptors and Recognition*, Series B, Volume 9)
Edited by S.J. Enna and H.I. Yamamura
Published in 1980 by Chapman and Hall, 11 New Fetter Lane,
London EC4P 4EE
© Chapman and Hall

1.1 INTRODUCTION

The potent neuroexcitatory effects of acidic amino acids were first described over 25 years ago (Hayashi, 1954). In the interim, through the sustained efforts of several neurophysiologic laboratories, evidence has accrued that glutamic acid and possibly aspartic acid may serve as excitatory neurotransmitters in the mammalian central nervous system (Curtis *et al.*, 1972; Curtis and Johnston, 1974; Krnjevic, 1974; McLennan, 1975). Prompted by these neurophysiologic observations, neurochemists over the last several years have attempted to identify neuronal pathways in the mammalian CNS that may utilize the acidic amino acids as their neurotransmitters; and neuropharmacologists have begun to explore interactions between drugs and the excitatory amino acids. An overview of this research suggests that the excitatory amino acids may play a fundamental role in brain function that is only beginning to gain wide appreciation. Thus, circumstantial evidence has implicated L-glutamic acid as the neurotransmitter for cortical pyramidal cells (Divak *et al.*, 1977; Lund-Karlsen and Fonnum, 1978), cerebellar granule cells (Young *et al.*, 1974) and primary sensory afferents (Johnson, 1972), in the mechanisms of action of sedatives and anticonvulsants (Richards and Smaje, 1976; MacDonald and Barker, 1979), and in the pathophysiology of certain neurodegenerative disorders (Perry *et al.*, 1977; Coyle, 1979).

An important technique for characterizing neurotransmitter function and the sites of drug action in brain is the receptor–ligand binding method. The criteria for inferring that a binding site represents a neurotransmitter receptor have been well established and rely heavily on the correlation between the rank order of potency of physiologically characterized agonists and antagonists and their efficacy in competing at the binding site (Cuatrecasas and Hollenberg, 1976; Burt, 1978). However, as will be discussed, the complexities of the neuronal interactions of the excitatory amino acids preclude facile correlations, and the absence of potent and specific inhibitors for their responses further undermine efforts to identify conclusively these receptors by biochemical techniques. Hence, the purpose of this review is to survey the neurophysiologic and neurochemical information on the action of excitatory amino acids that serves as the data base for receptor–ligand binding studies and, in this context, to assess critically the limited results obtained thus far with this method.

1.2 NEUROPHYSIOLOGY

1.2.1 Mammalian CNS

(a) Iontophoresis

Microiontophoresis has been used extensively to characterize the
neurophysiologic effects of excitatory amino acids at individual neurons or
at discrete loci on the invertebrate muscle (for review, see McLennan,
1970). With this technique, extremely fine cannulae, filled with drug
solutions and affixed to a recording electrode, are positioned near a
neuronal soma to record action potentials. The ionized drugs are expressed
from the cannula by an electrical current while alterations in neuronal
activity are measured. Although this is a powerful technique for eliciting
highly localized responses, it does suffer from important limitations with
regard to characterizing neurophysiologic effects of excitatory amino acids
(Davidson, 1976). Since the factors that determine the rate of egress of drug
from the cannula tip are complex and do not necessarily correlate with drug
concentration or current flow, potency comparisons among excitatory amino
acids and their analogues must be viewed with caution. Even when drug
concentration can be accurately controlled, both glia and neurons possess
avid sodium-dependent uptake mechanisms for several of the excitatory
amino acids that can variably affect the concentration of the agonist at
relevant receptor sites (Henn and Hamberger, 1971; Balcar and Johnston,
1972; Faive-Bauman *et al.*, 1974). Nearly all excitatory amino acids,
including their heterocyclic analogues, can be converted by decarboxylation
to neurophysiologically active derivatives with potent inhibitory effects that
can suppress excitatory responses; thus, L-aspartate can be decarboxylated to
form beta-alanine, L-glutamate to gamma-aminobutyric acid, ibotenate to
muscimol and quisqualic acid to quisqualamine (Johnston *et al.*, 1978; Evans
et al., 1978a). In addition, the acidic amino acids are to a varying degree
involved in other metabolic pathways that affect protein synthesis and
energy disposition in the cell (Berl *et al.*, 1970). Finally, responses produced
are highly dependent upon the cellular region of application of the agent;
there is a natural bias in mammalian CNS studies to place the electrode near
the neuronal soma to record brisk action potentials whereas relevant
excitatory receptors and excitatory inputs are thought to be concentrated on
the distal portions of the dendrites (Ransom *et al.*, 1977; Brookes, 1979).

(b) Excitatory cyclic analogues

In spite of these limitations, neurophysiologic studies have been facilitated
by the availability of several potent cyclical analogues and synthetic
derivatives of excitatory amino acids (Fig. 1.1). Many of these agents have
been isolated from biological sources including ibotenic acid, kainic acid,

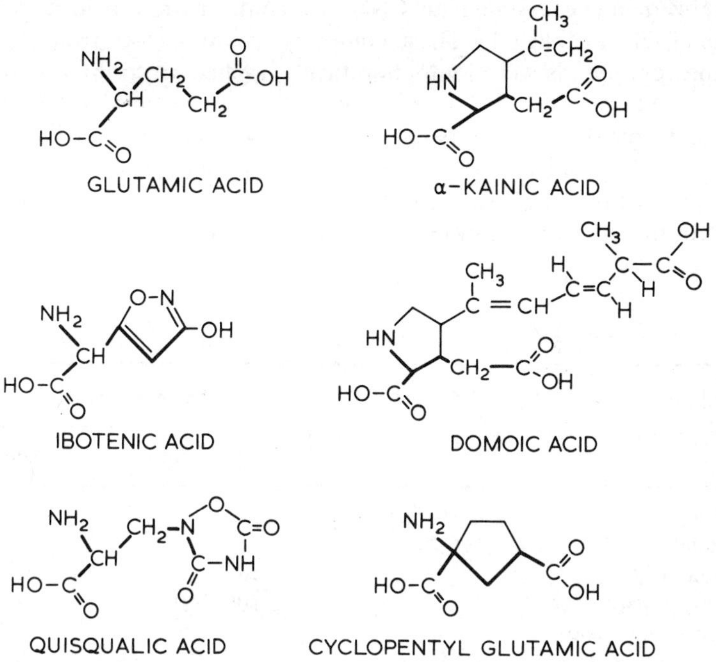

Fig. 1.1 Molecular structures of conformationally restricted analogues of glutamic acid. The glutamate sequence is indicated in each compound by the darker lines.

quisqualic acid and domoic acid (for review, see Takemoto, 1978). In addition, other compounds have been synthesized such as the cyclopentyl and cyclohexyl analogues of glutamic acid (McLennan and Wheal, 1978) and the alkyl derivative of aspartic acid, *N*-methyl-D,L-aspartic acid. Fortunately, these analogues appear to be poor substrates for the uptake and metabolic processes that act upon the parent amino acids. Because the prototypic excitatory amino acids – glutamic acid and aspartic acid – are highly flexible molecules capable of assuming a variety of conformations in solution, the rigid or restricted cyclical analogues serve as important tools for identifying the molecular orientation most suitable for interactions at the receptors. Finally, structural modifications of these compounds, which attenuate or eliminate their excitatory effects, have aided in clarifying molecular features critical for receptor activation.

(c) Structural activities
The structural–activity relationships for the excitatory effects of a large number of acidic amino acids and related compounds have been well

characterized in the mammalian CNS as recently reviewed in detail by
Watkins (1978) (Table 1.1). These comparisons are derived from studies in
which the compounds were iontophoretically applied on to interneurons in
the rat or cat spinal cord. In many cases, the results obtained in the
mammalian spinal cord have been correlated with the depolarization
of motor neurons in isolated frog or toad spinal segments produced by
superfusion with the agents. With this latter approach, drug concentration
can be controlled more accurately than with the iontophoretic technique.

Table 1.1 Excitatory potency of acidic amino acids and related compounds.

Compound	Relative potency*	
	Amphibian	Mammalian
Biological substances		
Quisqualic acid	416	22–90
Domoic acid	280	36–190
L-α-kainic acid	100–200	8–80
Dihydrokainic acid	—	0.06–0.8
D,L-ibotenic acid	22	2–7
β-N-oxalyl-α-β-diaminoproprionic acid	—	3–8
Dicarboxylic amino acids		
L-aspartic acid	0.8	0.7–1.0
D-aspartic acid	0.8–1.2	0.5
N-methyl-L-aspartic acid	5	1
N-methyl-D-aspartic acid	70	8
N-ethyl-D-aspartic acid	—	3
N-imino-methyl-D-aspartic acid	—	3
L-glutamic acid	1.0	1.0
D-glutamic acid	2.1–5.0	0.5
4-fluoro-glutamic acid	20	>1
2,4-diamino glutamic acid	5	—
Sulfur-containing amino acids		
L-homocysteic acid	15	1.0–1.4
D-homocysteic acid	20	2.8–5.0
D,L-homocysteic sulfinic acid	—	1.5
D,L-2-amino-4-thio sulfonyl butyric acid	8.3	4–11
L-S-sulfocysteine	6	3
L-cysteic acid	0.6	1
L-cysteine sulfinic acid	0.8	1

*The relative potencies of the compounds were determined by comparison with
L-glutamic acid. Values are based upon those tabulated by Watkins (1978).

From the large number of compounds examined, several structural features required for neuronal excitation can be deduced. Effective excitatory compounds invariably contain two separate acidic groups, which lose protons and become negatively charged at physiologic pH, and at least one basic group, which becomes positively charged at physiologic pH. In all compounds tested thus far, one of the acidic groups has been a carboxylic acid whereas the other group is capable of considerable variation and has included carboxyl, sulfinic, sulfonic, thiosulfonic, phosphonic and hydroxamic or other acidic alcoholic groups attached to an electron-withdrawing system. Invariably, the basic substituent has been an amino group. The acidic groups are optimally separated by a chain 3 to 4 carbons in length whereas the basic group is closely associated with one of the acidic groups. Structural modifications that reduce the ionizability of the acidic or basic substituents result in a marked attenuation in excitatory activity. Although the prototypic excitants – glutamic acid and aspartic acid – have minimal stereoselectivity in the vertebrate CNS (Biscoe *et al.*, 1976), their conformationally restricted analogues and alkylated derivatives often exhibit high degrees of stereoselectivity.

(d) Ionic effects

A detailed discussion of the ionic mechanisms responsible for the depolarizing effects of excitatory amino acids is beyond the scope of this review; nevertheless, since ion channels may be closely associated with, or allosterically interact with, their receptors, this issue is relevant to receptor binding studies. The depolarization caused by the acidic amino acids has generally, but not invariably, been associated with a marked increase in membrane conductance with variable effects on resistance, which is most compatible with an increase in membrane permeability to the sodium ion (Curtis *et al.*, 1972; Zieglgansberger and Puil, 1973; Hosli *et al.*, 1976). Some results that contradict this inference may reflect the fact that the amino acid has been iontophoresed close to the neuronal soma, some distance from the excitatory receptors on the distal portion of dendrites (Davidson, 1976). Notably, the sodium channels activated by the excitatory amino acids are distinct from the electrogenic sodium channels since the latter (Moore and Narahashi, 1967), but not the former, are blocked by tetrodotoxin (McIlwain *et al.*, 1969). However, increased sodium permeability may not be the only mechanism mediating the excitatory effects. Hence, Evans *et al.* (1977) have noted that the depolarizing action of L-homocysteate and D-glutamate are potentiated by sodium-deficient perfusion medium whereas the responses to other acidic amino acids were attenuated.

Neurochemical studies performed on mammalian brain slices incubated *in vitro* with excitatory amino acids including L-glutamate, L-aspartate,

L-homocysteate and *N*-methylaspartate substantiate the neurophysiologic conclusions that these agents depolarize neurons by increasing sodium permeability. Studies done by Bradford and McIlwain (1966), in which the uptake of sodium in cortical slices was correlated with membrane potential, have shown that the excitatory amino acids produced an increase in intraneuronal sodium that correlated closely, based on the Nerst equation, with membrane potential changes. The increase in sodium permeability resulted in an activation of the sodium–potassium-dependent ATPase which, with sustained exposure, caused a marked decrease in high-energy phosphates including ATP and phosphocreatine and substantial increases in inorganic phosphates, lactate, and cellular water (Harvey and McIlwain, 1968; Okamoto and Quastal, 1972; Cox *et al.*, 1977). However, kainic acid, except at quite high concentrations, did not affect ATP or cellular water but did increase intracellular sodium (Biziere and Coyle, 1978a).

(e) Antagonists
Specific antagonists play an essential role in characterizing the selectivity of the responses produced by iontophoretically applied neurotransmitters. Although several substances have been synthesized which interfere with amino acid-induced neuronal excitation, few if any exhibit a high degree of specificity. It should be noted that many of the potent neurotransmitter receptor blockers have been isolated from biological sources (atropine, bicuculline, alpha-bungarotoxin, etc.) and bear moieties that bind to portions of the receptor not evident on the basis of the structure of their receptor agonists. In contrast, most of the antagonists for excitatory amino acids have been synthesized through modifications of the basic structures of the excitatory amino acids themselves. Accordingly, it is not surprising that these agents, while competitive blockers, exhibit relatively poor differential affinity for the receptors. In addition, several of these antagonists directly inhibit neuronal activity when present in high concentrations; hence, inhibition must be distinguished from blockade of excitation (Altmann *et al.*, 1976; MacDonald *et al.*, 1977).

The specificity of the antagonism of acidic amino-induced depolarization has usually been determined by demonstrating that the agent is ineffective in blocking the excitatory effect of acetylcholine. Of the compounds tested, glutamate diethylester (Haldeman and McLennan, 1972), L-methionine, D,L-sulfoxamine (Curtis *et al.*, 1972), 5-6 dimethoxyaporphine (Hind and Kelley, 1975; Polc and Haefely, 1977), 2-amino-4-phosphonobutyric acid (Watkins *et al.*, 1977) and 3-amino-1-hydroxy-2-pyrrolidone (HA-966) (Curtis *et al.*, 1972) have been reported to exhibit greater effects against L-glutamate than against acetylcholine (Haldemen and McLennan, 1972); nevertheless, other studies have contradicted this degree of specificity (Altmann *et al.*, 1976; MacDonald *et al.*, 1977; Buu *et al.*, 1976).

Compounds more closely resembling aspartic acid such as D-alpha-aminoadipate, D-aminopimalate, D-alpha-aminosuberate and diaminopimelic acid appear to be selectively more potent in blocking the depolarization induced by *N*-methyl-D-aspartic acid than by that produced by glutamate (Biscoe *et al.*, 1978; Evans *et al.*, 1978b).

Based upon the clear-cut evidence for multiple types of receptors for other neurotransmitters (Snyder and Bennett, 1976), one might anticipate *a priori* that several receptors may mediate the excitatory effects of the structurally diverse acidic amino acids. For example, the considerable flexibility of glutamate allows the molecule to fold so that it closely resembles possible conformations of L-aspartate; however, L-aspartate, lacking one carbon in its chain cannot 'spread' the critical charged moieties to fit glutamate in an extended conformation. Comparative iontophoretic studies have revealed populations of neurons that exhibit differential sensitivity to L-aspartate and its alkyl derivative *N*-methyl-D-aspartate as compared to L-glutamate or its extended analogue, kainic acid (Duggan, 1974; McCulloch *et al.*, 1974). Based upon these observations and theoretical considerations, it has been suggested that at least two receptors may be involved (Buu *et al.*, 1976): one which recognizes glutamate and related compounds in the extended conformation and a second which recognizes aspartate or glutamate in a folded conformation.

Hall *et al.* (1979) have attempted to resolve this issue by comparing the neuroexcitatory potency and differential sensitivity to inhibitors of several conformationally restricted analogues of glutamic acid for which the intramolecular distances among the charged moieties have been defined (Table 1.2). Both L-glutamate and L-aspartate excite rat thalamic neurons although the former is two-fold more potent than the latter. Three glutamate analogues – kainate, *cis*-cyclopentyl glutamate and ibotenate – exhibit high excitatory potencies on thalamic neurons and share similar intramolecular distances between the alpha and omega carboxyl groups and the omega carboxyl group and the amino group. Notably, the distances between these charged substituents lie within the outer range for glutamate in the extended conformation but are well beyond that attainable by aspartate. Conversely, *trans*-cyclopentyl glutamate, which has an alpha to omega carboxyl gap similar to the other compounds but a separation between the omega carboxyl and the amino group comparable to aspartate, has an intermediate level of neuroexcitatory potency. Thus, on one extreme are the potent rigid neuroexcitants, capable of interacting with a receptor that can only recognize glutamate in the extended form, and on the other extreme is aspartate which is incapable of interacting with this receptor; an intermediate level of potency is found for glutamate, which can assume conformations fitting either the aspartate receptor or the more potent receptor for glutamate in an extended conformation.

While these results are compatable with two receptors, studies of the

Table 1.2 Conformational characteristics of excitatory amino acids.

Compound	Potency	$C_\alpha - C_\omega$ max	$C_\alpha - C_\omega$ min	$C_\omega - N$ max	$C_\omega - N$ min	GDEE	D-AA	Mg^{2+}
Kainate	10.6	5.1	4.4	4.6	3.0	1+	0	0
(±)Cis-1 amino-1,3 dicarboxycyclopentane	9.7		4.8		4.6	0	4+	—
Ibotenate	7.4	4.6	4.4	4.4	4.3	1+	4+	4+
N-methyl-D,L-aspartate	2.8	ND		ND		0	4+	4+
(±)Trans-1-amino-1,3 dicarboxycyclopentane	2.0		4.8		3.3	ND	ND	ND
D,L-homocysteate	1.8	ND		ND		0	4+	3+
L-glutamate	1.0	5.7	2.3	5.1	2.2	4+	1+	1+
D-aspartate	0.9	ND		ND		ND	ND	ND
L-aspartate	0.7	3.9	2.6	3.9	2.7	2+	2+	1+
D-glutamate	0.4	ND		ND		ND	ND	ND
(±)Cis-1-amino-1,3 dicarboxyhexane	0.1	5.0	2.4	4.3		ND	ND	ND

The excitatory potencies of the amino acids applied to rat thalamic neurons were determined relative to L-glutamate. The intramolecular distances between carboxy groups and the ω-carboxy group and the nitrogen were determined by computer models; the ranges are expressed in Å. The relative potency of glutamate diethylester (GDEE) and D-alpha-amino adipate (D-AA) were determined on thalamic neurons (Hall et al., 1979; McLennan and Lodge, 1979) whereas the antagonistic potency of magnesium ion (Mg^{2+}) was measured in frog spinal neurons (Evans et al., 1978b). ND = not done.

effects of receptor antagonists have undermined this simple dichotomy (Hall *et al.*, 1978; McLennan and Lodge, 1979). Glutamate diethylester was a consistently more potent antagonist of glutamate than of its extended, conformationally restricted analogues except quisqualate; nevertheless, it weakly antagonized L-aspartate. Conversely, the reputed L-aspartate antagonist, D-alpha-aminoadipate, was extremely effective in blocking the excitatory effects of *cis*-cyclopental glutamate and ibotenate, linear analogues of glutamate, as well as N-methyl-D,L-aspartate. Kainic acid stands alone in being relatively insensitive to both antagonists. In a similar vein, the studies of Evans *et al.* (1976) have shown that Mg^{2+} has differential inhibitory effects; notably, Mg^{2+} acted as a potent antagonist of N-methylaspartate but not of L-aspartate itself. These inconsistencies indicate that parceling of excitatory amino acid receptors in the mammalian central nervous system into aspartate-preferring or extended L-glutamate-preferring is an oversimplification (also, see Johnston, 1979). Furthermore, this issue is complicated by evidence for multiple site occupancy and co-operativity in amino acid-induced excitation (Constanti and Nistri, 1976).

(f) Excitatory amino acid pathways in mammalian brain

Neurotransmitter receptor distribution in brain generally correlates with the pattern of innervation for the neurons secreting the neurotransmitter (Snyder and Bennett, 1976). Thus, mapping of excitatory amino acid pathways in brain should aid in the identification and characterization of their postsynaptic receptors. The criteria for inferring that a neurotransmitter is utilized by a particular neuronal pathway include the demonstration that the neurotransmitter is synthesized, stored, released and taken up by the particular set of neurons and that drugs which block the postsynaptic effects of iontophoretically applied neurotransmitter also block the responses to the endogenous neurotransmitter released by the pathway in question (Florey, 1961; Phillis, 1966). Unfortunately, for the excitatory amino acids, these properties cannot be specifically associated with defined neuronal pathways in the same way possible for catecholaminergic, cholinergic or even GABAergic neurons.

The enzymes involved in the synthesis of glutamate or aspartate are not restricted to neurons, although future studies may reveal more selective localization of isozymal variants. As amino acids, glutamate and aspartate are contained in virtually all cell types and are involved in a variety of metabolic processes unrelated to their neurotransmitter role (Meister, 1965). Although certain neurons possess a sodium-dependent high-affinity transport process for glutamate and aspartate, a similar transport mechanism is also present on glial membranes (Henn *et al.*, 1974). Since nearly all neurons in the mammalian CNS can be depolarized by iontophoretic application of glutamate or aspartate (Curtis *et al.*, 1972), demonstration that neurons in the terminal field of a particular projection are sensitive to these amino acids can hardly be considered evidence of a specific innervation; however, it might be argued that excitatory amino acid innervation is so ubiquitous (e.g. the primary excitatory neurotransmitter) that nearly all cells do, in fact, receive such inputs (McLennan, 1975).

In the light of these problems, modified criteria must be applied to tentatively identify excitatory amino acid pathways in mammalian brain. Neurochemical evidence has been based upon the effects of selective lesions that destroy neuronal projections. If a neuronal pathway utilizes either glutamate or aspartate as its neurotransmitter, a selective reduction in the

Table 1.3 Putative glutamatergic and aspartergic pathways in mammalian brain.

Pathway	Transmitter	Neurochemistry	Neurophysiology
Cerebellar granule cells	Glu	(1–4)	(5)
Hippocampal perforant (cf: entorhinal cortex)	Glu	(6, 7)	(8)
Hippocampal commissural	Asp	(7)	(9)
Hippocampal-septal	Glu	(10–12)	(13)
Lateral olfactory tract	Glu	(14)	(15, 16)
Cortical-striatal	Glu	(17–19)	(20)
Primary sensory afferents	Glu	(21)	(22, 23)
Auditory nerve	Glu/Asp	(24, 25)	—
Cone photoreceptor	Asp	(26)	(27)

Several neuronal pathways or neuronal cell types in the mammalian CNS for which evidence suggests an excitatory amino acid neurotransmitter are listed. Neurochemical evidence is based upon the demonstration of selective reduction in the amino acid, its uptake system, or its release process whereas neurophysiologic evidence depends upon selective antagonism of postsynaptic effects by reputed excitatory amino acid antagonists.

Citations: (1) Young *et al.* (1974); (2) McBride *et al.* (1976a); (3) Valcana *et al.* (1972); (4) McBride *et al.* (1976b); (5) Stone (1979); (6) Nadler *et al.* (1976); (7) Nadler *et al.* (1978); (8) White *et al.* (1977); (9) Segal (1977); (10) Storm-Mathisen and Opsahl (1978); (11) Zaczek *et al.* (1979); (12) Fonnum *et al.* (1979); (13) DeFrance *et al.* (1973); (14) Harvey *et al.* (1975); (15) Bradford and Richards (1976); (16) Yamamoto and Matsui (1976); (17) Divac *et al.* (1977); (18) Kim *et al.* (1977); (19) Biziere and Coyle (1978b); (20) Spencer (1976); (21) Johnson (1972); (22) Dostrovsky and Pomeranz (1977); (23) Davies and Dray (1978); (24) Wenthold and Gulley (1978); (25) Wenthold (1978); (26) Neal (1976); (27) Wu and Dowling (1978).

level of endogenous glutamate or aspartate and a selective reduction in the activity of synaptosomal high-affinity uptake process for L-glutamate should occur in the region of terminal innervation following axotomy or destruction of the cell bodies of origin; conversely, presynaptic neurochemical markers for other systems innervating the region should remain unaffected.

However, the relatively high levels of L-glutamate and L-aspartate in the mammalian CNS create a substantial background that may adumbrate the neurotransmitter pool subject to reduction by lesion. Furthermore, the synaptosomal uptake system, which generally exhibits a more robust decrement as a result of lesion, cannot distinguish between aspartate or glutamate since they appear to share the same or nearly identical carrier (Balcar and Johnston, 1972; Cox and Bradford, 1978). However, Cotman and co-workers have developed evidence that regardless of which of the two radiolabeled amino acids is accumulated, upon depolarization the terminals release only the amino acid utilized by the neuron as its neurotransmitter (Nadler *et al.*, 1978). Neurophysiologic studies should demonstrate that excitatory amino acid antagonists specifically block the response produced by activation of the neuronal pathway in question. In addition, iontophoretic application of the excitatory amino acid should desensitize the postsynaptic receptors to their endogenous neurotransmitter. Based upon some or all of these criteria, several neuronal pathways in the mammalian brain have been implicated as using either glutamate or aspartate as their neurotransmitter (Table 1.3).

1.2.2 Invertebrates

(a) Neuromuscular junction
Considerable evidence has been developed that the excitatory neurotransmitter of the motor neurons innervating crustacean and insect striate muscles may be glutamic acid (Gershenfeld, 1973). The terminals of the motor neuron contain high concentrations of L-glutamate, actively accumulate glutamate (Iversen and Kravitz, 1968), release glutamate upon depolarization and the postsynaptic effects of the released neurotransmitter can be mimicked by iontophoretic application of glutamate (Kravitz *et al.*, 1970). The responsive sites are highly localized to the area of the muscle where excitatory junctional potentials can be recorded extracellularly. Furthermore, these receptors, which can be desensitized by prolonged application of glutamate, subsequently exhibit reduced sensitivity to the endogenous excitatory neurotransmitter. It should be noted, however, that the motor neurons also contain high concentrations of L-aspartic acid, which they release upon depolarization (McBride *et al.*, 1974). Although L-aspartate is a less effective excitant than glutamate at the crustacean neuromuscular junction (Kravitz *et al.*, 1970; Constanti and Nistri, 1979), it

potentiates the glutamate-induced depolarization (Shank and Freeman, 1975; Shank *et al.*, 1977). Recent evidence suggests that aspartate's potentiation results from its competitive inhibition of the uptake-inactivation of L-glutamate by the presynaptic terminal (Constanti and Nistri, 1978; McBurney and Crawford, 1979).

Several laboratories have probed the pharmacology of the excitatory receptors of the crayfish neuromuscular junction, relying heavily upon conformationally restricted analogues of glutamic acid including kainic acid and its derivatives, quisqualic acid and domoic acid. In contrast to the observations in mammalian brain, kainic acid has proved to be a weak, directly acting excitant at the crustacean neuromuscular preparation. When kainic acid was added to the medium perfusing the muscle, it was significantly less potent than L-glutamate in depolarizing the muscle membrane but potentiated the depolarizing action of L-glutamate (Shinozaki and Shibuya, 1974; Constanti and Nistri, 1976). Structural modifications of kainate that blocked the charged substituents on the molecule, e.g. acetylation of the ring nitrogen or esterification of the carboxyl groups, rendered the compound neurophysiologically inactive (Shinozaki and Shibuya, 1976). Thus, those portions of the molecule shared with glutamate are essential for activity. In addition, reduction of the isopropylene side-chain to form dihydrokainic acid or reversal of the plane of projection of the isopropylene side chain (alpha-allo-kainic acid) also attenuated its activity; accordingly, this part of the molecule plays an essential role in binding to the receptor. Consistent with this interpretation, domoic acid, which has a longer side-chain with an additional double bond and a carboxyl group (see Fig. 1.1), potentiated the glutamate-induced depolarization but also had direct excitatory effects (Shinozaki and Ishida, 1976). In contrast, quisqualic acid, which differs considerably in structure from kainate, proved to be exceedingly potent as a direct excitant but failed to potentiate the effects of glutamate.

Iontophoretic studies with kainic acid, in contrast to bath application, demonstrated that it was virtually inactive at glutamate sensitive receptors localized at the neuromuscular junction (Takeuchi and Ondoera, 1975; Daoud and Usherwood, 1975). When the effects of kainic acid were examined on the depolarization produced by iontophoretic application of glutamate to the 'hot spots', presumably the motor endplates, the potentiating effects of kainic acid were also negligible. The differential effects of kainate added to the perfusion medium with glutamate versus its iontophoretic application at sensitive sites has led to the suggestion that two different receptors may be involved in the response: a junctional receptor specifically sensitive to glutamic acid and insensitive to kainic acid and an extrajunctional receptor at which kainic acid can co-operatively interact with glutamic acid. Curiously, the depolarizing action of bath-applied quisqualic acid was inhibited by domoic acid or kainic acid in a noncompetitive manner (Shinozaki and Ishida, 1976). The differential effects of concanavalin A and dialtizam on glutamate potentials and excitatory junctional potentials have recently raised questions as to whether the endogenous transmitter of the crustacean motorneuron is, in fact, L-glutamate (Shinozaki and Ishida, 1979; Ishida and Shinozaki, 1980).

Wheal and Kerkut (1976) have found that at the abductor muscle of the walking leg of the hermit crab, kainic acid is two-fold more potent than L-glutamic acid in causing depolarization, whereas L-aspartic acid is approximately $\frac{1}{6}$ as potent; notably, ibotenic acid exhibits less than 0.005 per cent of the efficacy of L-glutamic acid. In contrast, kainic acid antagonized the depolarizing action of L-glutamate in the lobster walking limb (Shank and Freeman, 1976). Although the D- and L-forms of glutamic acid are nearly equipotent as neuroexcitants in the vertebrate CNS (Biscoe *et al.*, 1976), the D-forms have weak effects on the crustacean neuromuscular junction (Shank and Freeman, 1976; Constanti and Nistri, 1979). Two types of extrajunctional glutamate receptors have been identified on the extensor tibia muscle of the locust; a hyperpolarizing receptor which activates a chloride channel and is responsive to both glutamic acid and ibotenic acid and a depolarizing receptor, which is coupled to a sodium channel and possibly a potassium channel and is sensitive to glutamic acid but not to ibotenic acid (Cull-Candy, 1976; Clark *et al.*, 1979). In addition, glutamate acts at presynaptic receptors on the crustacean motorneuron terminals which may alter neurotransmitter release (Florey and Woodcock, 1968; Thieffry and Bruner, 1978).

(b) Invertebrate CNS

Neurophysiologists have also explored the effects of glutamic acid and related acidic amino acids in the central nervous system of molluscs, cephalopods and crustaceans. Because of the simplicity of their nervous systems and the large size of many of the neuronal somata, it is possible to impale specific, identified neurons with electrodes for intracellular recordings. Using these techniques, Miledi (1967; 1972) has demonstrated that extracellularly applied glutamate depolarized the giant axon in the squid stellate ganglia in the region of excitatory synapses. Discrete areas of high sensitivity corresponded to regions where the pre- and postsynaptic fibers came into close apposition. Notably, intracellular injection of glutamic acid did not affect the resting potential of the neurons, indicating that glutamate's action did not result from intracellular metabolic alterations but rather reflected interactions with receptors localized at the synaptic surface.

A variety of reproducible responses have been found for both L-glutamic acid and L-aspartate in the invertebrate central nervous system. These are linked to distinct ion channels and result in hyperpolarization due to increased permeability to chloride or depolarization resulting from increased permeability to sodium; less frequently, potassium-dependent channels have also been documented that result in slow hyperpolarization (Yarowsky and Carpenter, 1976; Eusebi *et al.*, 1978; Marder and Paupardin–Tritsch, 1978). These receptors share some features in common with those previously described on crustacean striate muscles. Kainic acid has been found to have weak depolarizing effects at the glutamate excitatory receptors but potentiates the action of L-glutamate. Conversely, quisqualic acid is up to 1000-fold more potent at the glutamate excitatory receptors but is weaker than glutamate at the inhibitory receptors (Walker, 1976). As noted for the extrajunctional inhibitory receptors on the crab muscle, ibotenic acid was a potent agonist at glutamate-sensitive receptors that cause hyperpolarization (Yokoi *et al.*, 1976).

(c) Summary

The results from neurophysiologic studies done in invertebrates suggest that considerable caution should be exercised in interpreting the effects of acidic amino acids in the mammalian CNS. First, the invertebrate studies have revealed important differences between receptors located at excitatory synapses and the extra-junctional receptors; and even at the neuromuscular junction, at least three distinct recognition sites can be detected (Gration *et al.*, 1979). The inherent problems of precisely defining the sites of iontophoretic application of acidic amino acids on mammalian CNS neurons preclude a firm distinction between junctional and extrajunctional receptors. Secondly, acidic amino acid receptors are not invariably associated with ion channels that result in depolarization; rather a variety of neurophysiologic responses occur with activation of these receptors in invertebrates. In a similar vein, while excitation predominates as the effect of acidic amino acids in the vertebrate CNS, inhibitory responses have occasionally been observed (Zieglgansberger and Puil, 1973; MacDonald and Nistri, 1977, 1978). Finally, the strikingly different neurophysiologic effects obtained with kainic acid, quisqualic acid, and ibotenic acid in the invertebrates considerably weakens the assumption that these agents activate a single class of glutamate receptors in the mammalian CNS.

1.3 EXCITOTOXINS

An indirect strategy for characterizing receptor-mediated effects of excitatory amino acids takes advantage of the neurotoxic potential of these agents. Lucas and Newhouse (1957) should be credited with the initial observation that intra-peritoneal administration of glutamic acid to neonatal rodents caused degeneration of neurons in the innernuclear layer of the retina. Subsequent studies indicated that in addition to the retina, neurons in the arcuate nucleus of the hypothalamus were also affected (Olney, 1969). Although the neurotoxic action of the acidic amino acids remained an enigma for over a decade, Olney *et al.* (1971) made the conceptual leap linking their neurotoxicity with their neuroexcitatory effects when they demonstrated that a variety of acidic amino acids were neurotoxic in proportion to their excitatory potency. The acute cytopathologic alterations produced by the acidic amino acids also correlated with their effects on ion permeability since shortly after treatment severe hydropic changes were first observed in the dendrites where excitatory amino acid receptors are concentrated (Olney, 1971). Furthermore, axons passing through the damaged hypothalamus were unaffected; consistent with this microanatomic specificity, mammalian axons are relatively insensitive to the depolarizing effects of acidic amino acids.

To avoid the interpretational complexities inherent in peripheral administration of these agents, such as the effects of metabolic transformation, blood–brain barrier, and hyperosmolarity, in more recent studies the neuroexcitants have been injected directly into the brain (Van Harreveld and Fifkova, 1971; Coyle and Schwarcz, 1976; McGeer and McGeer, 1976). Structural–activity studies have demonstrated a rough correlation between neuroexcitatory potency and neurotoxic effects of directly injected excitatory amino acids with the conformationally restricted analogues of glutamic acid exhibiting considerable activity; however, L-glutamic acid itself was minimally neurotoxic in remarkably high doses (Olney and de Gubareff, 1978b; Schwarcz *et al.*, 1978). Of the compounds examined, kainic acid has proved to be the most effective; whereas the neurophysiologically inactive derivatives (Shinozaki and Shibuya, 1976) of kainic acid including dihydrokainic acid, *N*-acetylkainic acid and kainate dimethylester lacked toxic effects (Schwarcz *et al.*, 1978).

Detailed morphologic and neurochemical studies have demonstrated that kainic acid caused degeneration of neurons with cell bodies near the site of injection but spared axons of passage or of termination from cell bodies distant from the injection site (Coyle and Schwarcz, 1976; Coyle *et al.*, 1978; Olney and de Gubareff, 1978a). Although virtually all CNS neurons are depolarized by the iontophoretic application of glutamate, neuronal sensitivity to the neurotoxic effects of kainic acid has proven quite variable. For example, a dose–response study in the dentate gyrus of the hippocampus has shown a hierarchy of neuronal vulnerability to kainic acid; in the order of decreasing sensitivity were CA3 pyramids > CA4 pyramids > CA1 pyramids > CA2 pyramids ≫ granule cells (Nadler *et al.*, 1978). When injected into the cerebellar cortex, kainic acid caused degeneration of all neuronal perikarya in several folia around the primary site of infusion except the granule cells; the granule cells, thought to be glutamatergic, synapse on the other vulnerable neuronal types but do not synapse upon each other (Herndon and Coyle, 1977). Thus, in the cerebellum, there appeared to be a correlation between glutamatergic innervation and neuronal vulnerability to kainic acid. Recent studies have shown that prior lesion of glutamatergic pathways to the striatum or the dentate gyrus of the hippocampus afforded considerable protection against the neurotoxic action of kainic acid in these regions (Biziere and Coyle, 1978b; Kohler *et al.*, 1978; McGeer *et al.*, 1978). Furthermore, anaesthetics and anticonvulsants, which interfere with excitatory neurotransmission, also attenuated the neurotoxic effects of kainic acid (Zaczek *et al.*, 1978). Taken together, these results suggest that the neurotoxic action of kainic acid may be indirect and may depend upon the functional integrity of excitatory afferents, which is consistent with its neurophysiologic action in the invertebrate (Shinozaki and Konishi, 1970).

In contrast to the variable sensitivity to kainic acid, preliminary data suggest that ibotenic acid, although less potent, caused a uniform sphere of neuronal degeneration following intracerebral injection (Schwarcz *et al.*, 1979). And differential sensitivity to *N*-methyl-D,L-aspartate as compared to L-glutamate has been reported in the arcuate nucleus of the hypothalamus (Olney *et al.*, 1979). Accordingly, further characterization of the neurotoxic effects of the various excitatory amino acids and their analogues may provide useful information concerning the function and distribution of excitatory amino acid receptors in the mammalian central nervous system.

1.4   CYCLIC NUCLEOTIDES AND EXCITATORY AMINO ACIDS

Characterization of receptor recognition sites by biochemical techniques have been greatly aided by methods that allow for the correlation between receptor occupancy and response. In an investigation of endogenous substances that activate adenylate cyclase, Shimizu *et al.* (1974) found that L-glutamate increased the levels of cyclic AMP by 80-fold in guinea-pig cortical slices incubated *in vitro*. This response appeared to be unique to brain and was not observed in peripheral organs such as liver or muscle. Other depolarizing agents like veratradine, which opens electrogenic sodium channels, ouabain, which inhibits sodium–potassium ATPase, and high potassium also produced marked elevation of the levels of cyclic AMP. Whereas the effects of these latter agents were partially reversed by calcium-free medium, indicative of their indirect mechanisms of action, the stimulation of adenylate cyclase by L-glutamate was not dependent upon Ca^{2+} in the medium. Furthermore, the response to L-glutamate could be distinguished from those of other adenylate cyclase systems such as norepinephrine, adenosine and histamine because their responses were additive with that of L-glutamate. The L-glutamate-induced activation of adenylate cyclase in the guinea-pig cortical slices exhibited several characteristics compatible with its mediation by an excitatory acidic amino acid receptor. Other excitatory amino acids including D-glutamic acid, L- and D-aspartic acids and L-cysteine sulfinate were also potent stimulators of cyclic AMP formation. Notably, ibotenic acid and kainic acid were nearly equipotent with L-glutamic acid; however, 2,4-diaminobutyrate blocked the effects of L-glutamate but not those of kainate and ibotenate (Shimizu *et al.*, 1975). The neurophysiologic specificity of the antagonistic effects of 2,4-diaminobutyrate has, however, been questioned (Bailey *et al.*, 1976).

Ferrendelli *et al.* (1974) demonstrated that L-glutamate increased the levels of cyclic GMP in mouse cerebellar slices incubated *in vitro*. Whereas GABA and glycine doubled the levels of cyclic GMP, L-glutamate caused an eleven-fold stimulation; the EC_{50} for L-glutamate was approximately 2 mM with maximal effects at 10 mM. Since neuronal guanylate cyclase is a soluble enzyme activated by an influx of Ca^{2+}, the Ca^{2+} dependence of the L-glutamate stimulation does not preclude a coupling of the excitatory receptors with the cyclase. The response to glutamate appeared to reflect its

Table 1.4 Effects of excitatory amino acids on cyclic nucleotides in cerebellar slices.

Compound	Per cent of control	
	Cyclic AMP	Cyclic GMP
Control	100	100
Glutamic acid (1 mM)	354	107
N-methyl aspartic acid (1 mM)	137	109
Homocysteic acid (1 mM)	402	122
Ibotenic acid (1 mM)	191	67
Kainic acid (1 mM)	4200	328
Dihydrokainic acid	115	131
Kainic acid + glutamate diethyester	4245	399
Kainic acid + EGTA and O–Ca^{2+}	88	59
Kainic acid + cocaine	3156	172
Kainic acid + theophylline	313	337
Kainic acid + adenosine deaminase	214	—

Slices of rat cerebellum were incubated with the various drugs; and the levels of endogenous cyclic AMP and cyclic GMP were measured (from Schmidt *et al.*, 1976).

depolarizing action since elevated potassium in the medium also produced a marked increase in the levels of cyclic GMP, which was not additive with the L-glutamate effect.

Schmidt and co-workers (1976, 1977) have expanded upon these initial observations by exploring the effects of kainic acid on the levels of cyclic AMP and cyclic GMP in rat brain slices incubated *in vitro* (Table 1.4). In the cerebellum, 1 mM kainic acid caused an 80-fold increase in the cyclic AMP levels and 3.5-fold increase in the cyclic GMP levels. This effect of kainic acid on cyclic nucleotides was highly restricted to the cerebellum since stimulation could not be elicited in cerebral cortex, hippocampus, hypothalamus or midbrain. Both cyclic AMP and cyclic GMP accumulations produced by kainic acid were blocked by calcium-free medium. Several excitatory amino acids produced a slight activation of adenylate cyclase that was 10- to 40-fold lower than that of kainic acid whereas these same compounds were ineffective in stimulating guanylate cyclase. Notably the neurophysiologically inactive derivative of kainic acid, dihydrokainic acid, was also ineffective in both systems. As suggested by the calcium dependence, the stimulation of cyclic AMP formation by kainic acid appeared to be indirect; since the kainate effect could also be inhibited by nearly 90 per cent by theophyline, 2-deoxyadenosine (both adenosine receptor antagonists) and adenosine deaminase, the stimulation likely reflected the release of adenosine by kainic acid. The cyclic GMP response, however, may be direct since adenosine antagonists did not inhibit it. In a recent *in vivo* study, Briley *et al.* (1979) have found that glutamate diethylester blocked the cyclic GMP accumulation in cerebellum stimulated by glutamate but not by kainic acid.

1.5 SPECIFIC BINDING OF GLUTAMIC AND ASPARTIC ACIDS

1.5.1 Invertebrates

Lunt (1973) published the first report in which specific binding of L-glutamic acid was examined with the express purpose of identifying an excitatory receptor. Because of the convincing evidence that glutamate acts as the neurotransmitter of motor neurons in the insect, he chose the thoracic muscles of the locust as his tissue source. Hydrophobic proteins were extracted from the muscle and solubilized with deoxycholate. On equilibrium dialysis, the extract exhibited saturable binding of L-glutamate with a K_D of approximately 0.5 μM and an apparent B_{max} of 170 nmol/mg protein; neither L-aspartic acid nor glutamine bound to a significant degree. The site was associated with membranes since aqueous extracts of the muscle did not bind either glutamate or glutamine. When the muscle membrane extract was chromatographed on Sephadex LH_{20} in the presence of [^{14}C]L-glutamic acid, the glutamate eluted in one major peak and a second minor peak in association of proteolipids; neither glutamine nor aspartate bound to these fractions. Since the locust neuromuscular junction is relatively insensitive to aspartate, the differential specificity for L-glutamic acid seemed compatible with the inference that the binding site may represent an excitatory receptor. However, the receptor density observed in equilibrium binding studies was unusually high, being several magnitudes greater than that reported for other neurotransmitter receptors in mammalian CNS or peripheral tissues (Bennett, 1978).

De Plazas and De Robertis (1974) utilized similar techniques to characterize a binding site for glutamate in hydrophobic proteins extracted from the striate muscle of the shrimp. This proteolipid, which was partially purified by chromatography on Sephadex LH_{20}, had an apparent K_D of 13 µM and B_{max} of 3.07 pmol/mg protein. The specific binding of L-glutamate was not inhibited by L-glutamine, L-aspartate or GABA; however, both glutamate diethylester and alpha methylglutamic acid caused substantial reductions in binding. Additional characterization of the binding sites with a wider range of conformationally restricted analogues and the demonstration of an anatomic distribution compatible with motor neuron receptors in the invertebrate would substantially strengthen conclusions about the receptor nature of these sites originally described by Lunt and De Robertis.

1.5.2 Mammalian CNS

Subsequently, De Robertis and De Plazas (1976) applied these methods to isolate hydrophobic proteins from cerebral cortical membranes of the rat. Crude synaptic membranes were prepared by differential centrifugation and extracted in chloroform–methanol. The extracts were chromatographed on Sephadex LH_{20} in the presence of [^{14}C]L-glutamic acid with chloroform and methanol as the eluant. A phosphoprotein peak that bound [^{14}C]L-glutamate was eluted with chloroform; this phosphoprotein was also eluted as a single peak when rechromatographed on a Merckogel OR-PVA 80 000 column and had different elution characteristics than a phosphoprotein which bound [^{14}C]GABA. Saturation isotherms revealed three different binding sites for L-glutamate with K_Ds of 0.3, 5 and 55 µM. The highest affinity site (0.3 µM) was markedly stereoselective for the L-isomer of glutamic acid and had a binding capacity of 530 pmol/mg protein. With a concentration ratio of inhibitor to ligand in excess of 100, glycine and glutamine produced slight inhibition, D,L-alphamethyl glutamic acid and nuciferine, a reported specific antagonist of glutamate-induced excitation, caused about 50 per cent inhibition of binding of L-glutamic acid whereas L-glutamate diethylester, a generally acknowledged glutamate receptor antagonist, inhibited binding by 65 per cent.

Utilizing a somewhat different approach, Michaelis *et al.* (1974) have identified specific binding sites for L-glutamate in rat brain. Synaptic membranes were isolated by subcellular fractionation monitored by electron microscopy and enzymatic markers. The membranes were solubilized by treatment with Triton X-100 (0.5 per cent) and the binding of L-glutamate was measured by equilibrium dialysis. Specific binding sites for L-glutamate were markedly enriched in the synaptic membranes as compared to mitochondrial, microsomal and nuclear membrane subfractions. The pH optimum for binding was 8.0. Low concentrations of Ca^{2+} (0.5 mM) enhanced specific binding; however, Mg^{2+} was ineffective. The specific binding was inversely proportional to the ionic strength of the incubation medium. Saturation isotherms revealed two binding sites: a higher affinity site with a K_D of 18 nM and a B_{max} of 4.4 nmol/mg protein and a lower affinity site with a K_D of 2.1 µM. Additional kinetic analysis suggested positive co-operativity between the two sites with Hill coefficients of 1.6 to 2.6. The excitatory amino acids cysteine sulfinic acid, homocysteic acid and L-aspartic acid inhibited the specific binding of L-glutamate by 40 to 60 per cent at a concentration of competitor two-fold greater than ligand. Notably, the inhibitory amino acids glycine and beta-alanine produced only modest inhibition; however, GABA proved to be a potent antagonist although Dixon plots indicated that GABA's effect was noncompetitive. Whereas neurophysiologically inactive substances such as *N*-acetylaspartate, glutamine and amino oxyacetic acid did not compete at the binding site, the glutamate receptor blocker glutamate diethylester exerted mild inhibition.

The solubilized receptor was sensitive to inactivation by prior treatment with trypsin, pronase, beta-glucosidase, and phospholipase C. From these results, it was inferred that the binding site was a glycoprotein interacting closely with phospholipids. In support of this interpretation, pre-incubation of the solubilized receptor with the plant lectin concanavalin A, which binds to certain glycosides, completely inhibited the specific binding of glutamate. This property was exploited to further purify the binding site by affinity chromatography with concanavalin A linked to Sepharose (Michaelis, 1975). The purified glycoprotein on SDS gel electrophoresis had a molecular weight of 13 880 daltons; and the protein band reacted with periodic acid–Schiff stain. Notably, concanavalin A also alters the neurophysiologic effects of L-glutamate at the crustacean muscle (Shinozaki and Ishida, 1979). In contrast to the Triton solubilized binding site, the purified protein exhibited a single class of binding sites with a K_D of 0.85 µM and a B_{max} of 65 nmol/mg protein. Competitive inhibition studies indicated that the excitatory amino acids L-aspartic acid, D,L-homocysteic acid and D-L-cysteine sulfinic acid as well as the antagonist glutamate diethylester were relatively potent competitors of the specific binding of L-glutamate whereas D-glutamic acid and the inhibitory amino acids glycine, beta-alanine and GABA produced negligible inhibition. Based upon the fact that sodium azide profoundly inhibited binding, Michaelis (1979) recently developed evidence that the protein contains two atoms of iron and two atoms of sulfur that may be directly involved in the recognition site.

Michaelis and co-workers have also demonstrated in a partially purified synaptosomal membrane fraction specific binding of L-glutamate which shares many properties with the Triton solubilized receptor. Thus, higher (K_D 0.2 mM) and lower (K_D 1 mM) affinity sites, which exhibited positive co-operativity (Hill coefficients = 2.6 to 3.0), could be observed in the intact membranes. Furthermore, the membrane binding sites were sensitive to pre-incubation with proteases and lipases as well as exposure to concanavalin A. Recently this group has reported that treatment with ethanol *in vitro* as well as *in vivo* alters the synaptic membrane binding site for L-glutamate (Michaelis *et al.*, 1978). *In vitro*, ethanol concentrations from 5 to 50 mM caused an increase in specific binding of L-glutamate whereas concentrations of ethanol above 50 mM result in a progressive decrease in binding. With chronic administration of ethanol to rats, there was an increase in the specific binding of glutamate in synaptic membranes that appeared to reflect an increase in the number of sites with no apparent change in K_D. However, the complex nature of the saturation isotherms with Hill coefficients ranging from 2.4 to 4.9 precluded firm conclusions about the kinetic basis of the alterations. After discontinuation of ethanol, glutamate binding in the synaptic membranes from the rats gradually returned to the control state. Behavioral pharmacologic correlates of these alterations have been provided by studies demonstrating that the glutamate receptor antagonist, glutamate diethylester, attenuated seizures in mice produced by acute alcohol withdrawal and that ethanol-dependent mice were more sensitive to the seizure-inducing effects of peripherally administered kainic acid (Freed and Michaelis, 1978).

Roberts was among the first to describe specific binding of L-glutamate in mammalian brain neuronal membranes (Roberts, 1974). In a recent publication, this site has been extensively characterized in the synaptic membranes prepared from rat cerebellum (Foster and Roberts, 1978). Specific binding was measured by a rapid centrifugation technique, in which membranes were incubated with nanomolar concentrations of L-[^{3}H]glutamic acid in the presence or in the absence of unlabeled L-glutamate (1 mM) to distinguish specific from nonspecific binding. Optimal specific binding was obtained at pH 7.5 at 37° C; prior freezing of the tissue caused a 90 per cent reduction in specific binding but did not affect the nonspecific binding. The binding sites were markedly enriched in the synaptosomal membranes with a four- to eight-fold lower concentration in

purified myelin and mitochondrial membranes. Nevertheless, membranes
prepared from lung, kidney and striate muscle specifically bound from 12 to
30 per cent of that found in the cerebellum. Saturation isotherm revealed a
single population of binding sites in the cerebellar synaptic membranes with
a K_D of 744 nM and a binding capacity of 73 pmol/mg protein.

An extensive structural activity analysis of inhibitors of specific glutamate
binding in the cerebellum provided convincing evidence that the site may
represent an excitatory glutamate receptor (Table 1.5). Next to glutamate
itself, the two most potent displacers were ibotenic acid and quisqualic acid;
notably, neither kainic acid nor dihydrokainic acid significantly inhibited

Table 1.5 Inhibition of the specific binding of [^{3}]-L-glutamate
to rat cerebellar synaptic membranes.

Compound	$IC_{50}(\mu M)$
L-glutamic acid	4.8
D,L-ibotenic acid	8.1
D,L-quisqualic acid	8.4
D,L-homocysteic acid	10.8
Trans-1-amino-1,3-dicarboxycyclopentane	17.9
Cis 1-amino-1,3-dicarboxycyclopentane	18.5
D,L-2-amino-4-phosphonobytyric acid	25.6
D,L-α-amino adipic acid	26.3
D-glutamic acid	28.8
L-aspartic acid	42.1
L-glutamate-8-hydroxamate	65.9
L-glutamine	116.8
D-aspartic acid	138.0
L-glutamate diethylester	1000
L-methionine-D,L-sulfoximine	>1000
Kainic acid	>1000
Dihydrokainic acid	>1000
N-methyl-D,L-aspartic acid	>1000
HA-966	>1000

Cerebellar synaptic membranes were assayed for specific bonding of [^{3}H]L-
glutamic acid (0.8 μM) in the presence of a wide range of concentrations
of the agents which inhibit specific binding by 50 per cent. Results taken from
Foster and Roberts (1978).

specific binding at a concentration 1200-fold greater than the ligand. The conformationally restricted analogues of glutamic acid, *trans*-1-amino-1,3-dicarboxycyclopentane and *cis*-1-amino-1,3-dicarboxy-cyclopentane were approximately four-fold less potent than L-glutamate. Since the results with these conformationally restricted analogues suggested that the receptor recognized glutamate in the extended form, it is not surprising that D- and L-aspartate and N-methyl-D,L-aspartate were poor inhibitors. The glutamate receptor antagonists 2-amino-4-phosphonobutyric acid and D,L-alpha amino adipic acid were approximately five-fold less potent than L-glutamate whereas glutamate diethylester and HA-966 were relatively weak inhibitors of binding. The site had only a seven-fold preference for L- as compared to the D-stereoisomer of glutamic acid. Finally, the fact that hydroxamates of glutamate and aspartate, potent inhibitors of the presynaptic transport process, were relatively ineffective antagonists argued against the possibility that the binding site represented a carrier for the sodium-dependent, high-affinity uptake process.

Biziere *et al.* (1980) have also examined the specific binding of [^{3}H]L-glutamic acid to crude membrane preparations isolated from rat forebrain using the centrifugation technique. Focusing on low concentrations of the ligand, they demonstrated two populations of binding sites in saturation isotherms with K_Ds of approximately 11 and 80 nM. Hill plots did not uncover co-operative interactions between the two sites. Displacement studies revealed a moderate degree of stereospecificity for the L-form of glutamic acid; other neuroexcitants such as L-aspartic, D,L-homocysteic and L-cysteine sulfinic acids were relatively potent competitors as was also the case for the conformationally restricted analogue *cis*-1-amino-1,3-dicarboxycyclopentane. D-aspartic and N-methyl-D,L-aspartic acids exhibited negligible activity, and the nonexcitatory analogues L-cysteine, and L-homocysteine thiolactone were also poor competitors. In contrast to the report of Foster and Roberts (1978), neither quisqualic acid nor ibotenic acid were effective inhibitors; also kainic acid and dihydrokainic acid exhibited negligible affinity for the site. In terms of potency of glutamate receptor blockers, D,L-alpha aminoadipic acid was three-fold more effective than D,L-1-amino-4-phosphonobutyric acid whereas L-glutamate diethylester was relatively weak. These binding sites had an uneven distribution in brain with cortical regions and the striatum having the highest concentration (Table 1.6).

These binding sites were unlikely to represent a carrier for L-glutamate since the hydroxamates of glutamate and aspartate were poor inhibitors of specific binding (Balcar and Johnston, 1972). In support of this interpretation, prior lesion of the cortico-striatal glutamatergic pathway, which reduced synaptosomal high-affinity uptake of glutamate in the

Table 1.6 Regional distribution of specific binding sites for [³H]kainic acid and [³H]L-glutamic acid in rat brain.

Region	[³H]kainic acid	[³H]L-glutamic acid
Parietal cortex	22 ± 2	20 ± 2
Frontal cortex	17 ± 2	22 ± 1
Hippocampus	18 ± 2	26 ± 2
Striatum	27 ± 2	16 ± 2
Thalamus	—	8 ± 1
Cerebellum	12 ± 1	6 ± 1
Pons-medulla	1 ± 0.2	5 ± 1
Hypothalamus	10 ± 1	5 ± 1

Results have been taken from Coyle (1979) and Biziere *et al*. (1980). Specific binding was measured in the presence of 50 nM [³H]kainic acid or 30 nM [³H]L-glutamic acid, and values are expressed in terms of fmol/mg tissue.

striatum by 40 per cent, did not affect the specific binding of [³H]L-glutamate in striatal membranes. In contrast, destruction of striatal intrinsic neurons by prior lesion with kainic acid caused a 45 per cent reduction in the specific binding of [³H]L-glutamate, a reduction comparable to that observed for other neurotransmitter receptor sites after striatal kainate lesion (Coyle, 1979). Thus, the binding sites appeared to be concentrated upon neurons within the striatum and were unlikely to have a presynaptic localization on excitatory afferents.

Little has been published on the specific binding of L-aspartate to putative excitatory receptors except for a brief report by De Robertis and De Plazas (1976). Using techniques similar to that for isolating the proteolipid binding site for L-glutamate, chloroform–methanol extracts of rat brain membrane preparations were separated by column chromatography on Sephadex LH–20. A peak of protein was eluted with chloroform that specifically bound [¹⁴C]L-aspartic acid; saturation studies revealed three apparent binding sites with dissociation constants of 0.2, 10 and 50 μM and binding capacities of 2.8, 132 and 617 nmol/mg protein, respectively. Cross-binding studies suggested that L-glutamate and L-aspartate were binding to different proteolipids. Whereas L-glutamate diethylester, alpha methyl glutamic acid and nuciferine were relatively potent inhibitors of L-glutamate binding, they were much weaker at the L-aspartate site; a concentration of kainic acid that inhibited the specific binding of L-glutamate by 50 per cent had no effect on the L-aspartate site. In contrast, *N*-methyl-D-L-aspartic acid inhibited the binding of L-aspartate but did not effect the binding of L-glutamate.

1.5.3 Summary

A synthesis of the information derived from these studies on the specific binding of acidic amino acids is confounded by critical differences in the methods used among the various laboratories. Clearly, the invertebrate neuromuscular junction serves as an excellent tissue source for characterization and isolation of a population of neurophysiologically well-defined glutamate receptors; however, the limited studies done with this preparation, while promising, lack sufficient information about the structural–activity relationships of other agonists and antagonists and cellular localization to conclude with confidence that the binding sites represent excitatory receptors. With regard to studies done in the mammalian CNS, a family of sites with affinity constants ranging from 10 nM to 1 mM have been described depending upon assay conditions. It is noteworthy that in most cases the affinity of the binding sites for glutamate are rather low (> 0.5 μM) in contrast to the nM affinities described for other neurotransmitter receptors (Bennett, 1978; Burt, 1978); nevertheless, this lower affinity is entirely compatible with the concentrations neurophysiologically required to produce excitation. Although structural–activity relations, regional and subcellular distribution and pharmacologic characteristics support the inference that some of these sites may represent excitatory receptors, important differences among results obtained by the various laboratories makes it difficult to determine whether separate or related sites are being studied.

1.6 SPECIFIC BINDING OF [^{3}H]KAINIC ACID

Because of the multiplicity of sites with which L-glutamate interacts, excitatory amino acid receptor characterization would be simplified by the use of conformationally restricted analogues that selectively bind to subsets of the glutamate receptors. Furthermore, neurophysiologic evidence indicates that these analogues are considerably more potent than L-glutamate; their higher affinity for receptors should allow for a more stable ligand–receptor complex amenable to isolation and characterization. The only conformationally restricted analogue of glutamate studied thus far with receptor-binding techniques has been [^{3}H]kainic acid. It should be noted that many of the studies with this ligand have been prompted by the assumption that kainic acid is a specific agonist for glutamate receptors in the mammalian CNS; this belief, however, does not receive much support from the neurophysiologic studies reviewed above. Nevertheless, because of its marked potency and specificity of the action, kainic acid represents a useful ligand for characterizing a subset of receptors involved in excitatory neurotransmission in the mammalian CNS.

Simon *et al.* (1976) were the first to publish a detailed study on the specific binding of [³H]kainic acid to synaptic membranes from rat brain; subsequently a number of other reports have appeared which have confirmed and expanded upon these original observations (Johnston *et al.*, 1979; Schwarcz and Fuxe, 1979; Vincent and McGeer, 1979). Most investigators have found a single population of binding sites with an apparent K_D of 40 to 60 nM; but, a second higher affinity binding site with a K_D of 3 to 5 nM has also been recently described (Beaumont *et al.*, 1979; London and Coyle, 1979b). The binding sites are concentrated in brain and virtually undetectable in membranes isolated from peripheral tissues. In a study of the subcellular distribution of the binding site in brain, it was found to be markedly enriched in the crude synaptosomal membranes and relatively deficient in other fractions (Simon *et al.*, 1976). The binding sites exhibit an unequal regional distribution in rat brain with corpus striatum having the highest concentration, cerebral cortex somewhat lower, intermediate levels in the cerebellum and lowest levels in the brainstem regions including hypothalamus, medulla and pons (Table 1.7).

At the K_D 50 nM binding site, aside from authentic kainic acid, quisqualic acid is the most potent displacer; L-glutamic acid follows with 20-fold lower affinity than kainic acid itself (Table 1.7). The receptor is highly

Table 1.7 Affinities of various substances for [³H]kainic acid receptor binding sites in rat forebrain.

Compound	K_I at high-affinity receptor (µM)	K_I at low-affinity receptor (µM)
Kainic acid	0.001	0.013
Quisqualic acid	0.023	0.255
L-glutamic acid	0.063	0.722
Ibotenic acid	3.30	35.7
Dihydrokainic acid	6.60	3.15
D,L-homocysteic acid	7.12	87.2
L-glutamine	19.4	6.4
D-glutamic acid	155.0	42.0
L-glutamate diethyl ester	>100	>100
N-methyl-D,L-aspartic acid	>100	>100
2-amino-4-phosphonobutyric acid	>100	>100
Nuciferine	>100	>100

Values taken from London and Coyle (1979b).

stereospecific with D-glutamic acid having approximately a 2000-fold lower affinity. Notably, another potent neuroexcitant, ibotenic acid is also a weak competitor of the binding site. L- and D-aspartic and N-methyl-D,L-aspartic acids have negligible affinity for the receptor. The inactive derivative of kainic acid, dihydrokainic acid, has a 250-fold lower affinity for the receptor site. A variety of other amino acids and neurotransmitters with neurophysiologic effects unrelated to glutamate are ineffective as inhibitors of specific binding.

The low affinity of dihydrokainic acid for the receptor is compatible with the neurophysiologic and neurotoxocologic observations that this derivative is inactive (Shinozaki and Shibuya, 1976; Schwarcz *et al.*, 1978). These results suggest that the isopropylene side-chain of kainic acid plays a fundamental role in its binding to the receptor site, a portion of the molecule that has no homology in the structure of L-glutamic acid. Detailed inhibition studies with L-glutamic acid, D-glutamic acid and dihydrokainic acid on the specific binding of [^{3}H]kainic acid to cerebellar membranes, which possess only the 50 nM K_D site, have revealed flat displacement curves with Hill coefficients of 0.5; in contrast, unlabeled kainic acid displaced [^{3}H]kainic acid according to mass action kinetics with a Hill coefficient of 1.0 (London and Coyle, 1979a). These results are compatible either with negative co-operativity between dihydrokainic, D- and L-glutamic acids and the kainic acid binding site or with the kinetics of multiple site interactions (DeLean *et al.*, 1979).

As noted above, a second higher affinity site was defined by saturation isotherms with an apparent K_D of 3 to 5 nM in rat brain (London and Coyle, 1979b). This second site did not appear to be an artifact of the radioligand since it has been observed with separate batches of [^{3}H]kainic acid of different specific radioactivities and was apparent on saturation isotherms with [^{3}H]kainic acid as well as competitive displacement curves with unlabeled kainic acid. Calculation of the equilibrium dissociation constant for the high affinity site from the rates of association and dissociation resulted in a similar value. Because [^{3}H]kainic acid dissociates from the lower affinity (K_D 50 nM) binding site very rapidly, the high-affinity site can be studied independently of the low affinity by occlusion of low-affinity sites with an excess of unlabeled kainic acid added at the end of incubation (London and Coyle, 1979b). Although there are many similarities in the characteristics of these two sites, aside from their ten-fold difference in apparent K_Ds, certain disparities were noteworthy. For example, dihydrokainic acid, L-glutamine and D-glutamic acid were relatively weaker competitors at the higher affinity site than at the lower affinity site. The higher affinity site also had a different regional distribution in brain, being concentrated primarily in striatum and cortical regions and virtually absent from the cerebellum and medulla-pons.

If the binding sites for [³H]kainic acid represent the receptor mediating its neurophysiologic effects, then they should decrease as a result of neuronal degeneration produced by intracerebral injection of kainic acid. Direct injection of kainic acid into the rat corpus striatum caused a profound degeneration of neurons with cell bodies in the region. Although receptor binding for [³H]kainic acid was unaffected 1 week after lesion, by 4 to 7 weeks after injection, receptor binding for [³H]kainic acid was reduced by 60 to 80 per cent (Beaumont *et al.*, 1979; Biziere and Coyle, 1979b; London and Coyle, 1979b). This delayed and gradual decrease in receptor binding sites following a kainate lesion is compatible with the slow clearance of postsynaptic specialization enriched with receptors that has been documented by electron microscopic studies (Coyle *et al.*, 1978). Intraocular injection of kainic acid produced a highly selective pattern of degeneration in the chick retina that affected primarily the interneurons in the innernuclear layer while sparing rods, cones, ganglion cells and glia (Schwarcz and Coyle, 1977). 7 days after the intraocular injection of kainic acid, the specific binding of [³H]kainic acid to retinal membranes was reduced by 75 per cent (Biziere and Coyle, 1979b). This decrement indicates that the binding sites are highly concentrated on retinal interneurons vulnerable to kainic acid but are relatively deficient on other cellular types in the retina that survive the kainic acid lesion. The indirect mechanism of kainate's neurotoxicity has prompted the suggestion that kainic acid may exert its effects at presynaptic receptors on glutamatergic afferents. Lesion studies of defined glutamatergic pathways, however, have not demonstrated a sustained or marked decrease in specific binding sites for [³H]kainic acid in the affected terminal field (Biziere and Coyle, 1979b; Henke and Cuenod, 1979).

Ontogenetic studies in the brain have demonstrated that several well-characterized neurotransmitter receptors increase in density in a manner that correlates with synaptic maturation (Coyle, 1977). A developmental study of the specific, high affinity binding of [³H]kainic acid to membranes prepared from rat striatum indicated that binding is quite low during the first week after birth but developed rapidly between 10 and 28 days after birth (Campochiaro and Coyle, 1978). The phase of increasing kainate receptor binding corresponded with the period of intense synaptogenesis in the striatum. More importantly, striatal neuronal vulnerability to local injection of kainic acid developed in concert with the receptor. Thus, kainic acid injected into the striatum of the 7-day-old rat was virtually devoid of neurotoxicity whereas an adult pattern of sensitivity appeared by 21 days of age when the receptor binding sites had achieved 70 per cent of adult levels. These ontogenetic studies provide additional evidence that the binding sites for [³H]kainic acid mediate its effects in mammalian CNS.

Since neurophysiologic and neurotoxocologic studies indicate that kainic acid has potent effects in species ranging from insects to primates, it seems likely that its receptors have a broad phylogenetic distribution (Table 1.8). In fact, an uneven phylogenetic distribution of the ^{3}H-kainate receptors has been found with relatively low levels in primitive species such as hydra, at one extreme, and in advanced species such as mammals, at the other extreme (London *et al.*, 1980). At the intermediate levels including fish, amphibians and avians, high levels of specific binding of ^{3}H-kainate have been found in the nervous system. Kinetic studies have revealed similarities in the binding sites in amphibians and avians to those described in mammalian brain. Thus, dihydrokainic acid and D-glutamic acid have relatively low affinities for the receptors and both stereoisomers of glutamic acid and dihydrokainic acid exhibit flat displacement curves with Hill coefficients of approximately 0.5. Since the concentration of binding sites is nearly 100-fold greater in the frog brain than in mammalian brain, these lower species may serve as useful sources of receptor for additional characterization and possibly for purification.

Table 1.8 Phylogenetic distribution of the specific binding sites for [^{3}H]kainic acid.

	Region	fmol/mg protein
Hydra	Whole organism	609 ± 195
Sea anemone	Whole organism	0
Planaria	Head ganglia	68 ± 27
Earthworm	Head ganglia	271 ± 29
Crayfish	Head ganglia	44 ± 17
Cockroach	Head ganglia	161 ± 86
Hagfish	Whole brain	27 ± 13
Spiny dogfish	Cerebellum	77 250 ± 8 550
Goldfish	Whole brain	6 560 ± 20
Frog	Whole brain	94 100 ± 23 400
Chicken	Cerebellum	2 900 ± 168
Rat	Cerebellum	210 ± 38
Man	Cerebellum	224 ± 18

Specific binding of [^{3}H]kainic acid was measured in the presence of 10 nM concentration of ligand; results are expressed in terms of fmol specifically bound per mg membrane protein. Values are taken from London *et al.* (1980).

1.6.1 Summary

In contradistinction to the studies done in mammalian CNS with [^{3}H]glutamate, there is remarkable concurrence among the various laboratories concerning the characteristics of the specific binding sites for [^{3}H]kainic acid. These studies have demonstrated that the binding is localized in brain, enriched in synaptosomal fractions and highly associated with neurons vulnerable to the neurotoxic action of kainic acid. Structural–activity studies indicate that the binding site exhibits a higher affinity for kainate than for L-glutamate, has marked stereospecificity for the L-isomer of glutamate unlike the recognition site that mediates the excitatory effects of glutamic acid in mammalian brain, and is relatively insensitive to a variety of antagonists that inhibit the excitatory effects of acidic amino acids. Furthermore, anomalous kinetics of inhibition by dihydrokainate and the stereoisomers of glutamate emphasize the importance of isopropylene side-chain, which has no homology in glutamic acid. These characteristics seem incompatible with the conclusion that this ligand labels the receptors mediating the excitatory effects of glutamate in mammalian CNS. What remains to be clarified is whether this receptor site represents a subset of excitatory amino acid receptors or rather the recognition site for some other endogenous substance.

1.7 CONCLUSION

The value of a review of an area of research in its early stages of development, as is the case for binding studies of the excitatory amino acids receptors, lies not so much in summarizing what has been done but rather in defining issues needing further investigation. Progress in characterizing these receptors depends heavily upon a further elucidation of receptor specificity and micro- and macrotopology in the brain as well as identification of excitatory amino acid pathways. But in the more restricted sense, the following issues merit particular attention.

First, the absence of potent and specific antagonists for acidic amino acid-induced neuronal excitation has been a major impediment in the neurophysiologic and neurochemical characterization of their receptors. While the modification of their structure serves as an important approach for developing potential antagonists, this strategy has achieved limited success thus far. Based upon characteristics of other neurotransmitter antagonists, it would seem that screening biological sources for neuroexcitant antagonists would be a more successful way of identifying potent compounds that interact with sites on the receptor not apparent from agonist studies. Since glutamate is most likely the neurotransmitter at the insect neuromuscular junction, biological substances with insecticidal activity might be particularly promising. In the light of the fundamental role of excitatory amino acids in mammalian CNS, identification of potent antagonists is not simply of heuristic interest since these compounds would likely have pharmacologic activity as sedatives, muscle relaxants and anticonvulsants.

Secondly, there is a definite need to increase the types of radiolabeled, conformationally restricted analogues of excitatory amino acids for receptor–ligand binding studies. Although some critics may complain that the number of 'receptors' is proliferating in proportion to the radioligands available, neurophysiologic data provide convincing evidence that quisqualic acid, ibotenic acid, *N*-methyl-aspartic acid and *cis*-cycloglutamic acid interact with subsets of excitatory receptors. The higher affinity and conformational rigidity of these compounds indicate their superiority over [³H]L-glutamic acid or [³H]aspartic acid as ligands in receptor binding studies.

Thirdly, advantage should be taken of the coupling of certain excitatory amino acid receptors with brain cyclase systems. Because of the immediate depolarizing action of acidic amino acids, it is unlikely that these receptor-linked cyclases serve as the primary transducers of their excitatory effects; and their function remains to be identified. Nevertheless, the availability of a system in which the consequences of excitatory amino acid receptor occupancy can be correlated with a biochemically defined response offers an important opportunity for identifying *in vitro* agents that interact with these receptors.

Finally, because the neurophysiologic effects of glutamate have been most clearly defined at the invertebrate neuromuscular junction, the motor end plate is the logical starting point for rigorous characterization of glutamate receptors. In addition, the preliminary evidence has revealed a high concentration of [³H]kainic acid receptors in fish and amphibian CNS. Thus, as electroplax has played a major role in the study of the nicotinic acetylcholine receptor, submammalian species should be exploited as sources rich in excitatory amino acid receptors, suitable for isolation, purification and detailed biochemical analysis.

REFERENCES

Altmann, H., Ten Bruggencate, G., Pickelmann, P. and Steinberg, R. (1976), *Pflugers Arch.*, **364**, 249–255.
Bailey, P.A., Phillis, J.W. and Sastry, B.S.R. (1976), *Gen. Pharmacol.*, **7**, 421–425.
Balcar, V.J. and Johnston, G.A.R. (1972), *J. Neurochem.*, **19**, 2657–2666.
Beaumont, K., Maurin, Y., Reisine, T.D., Fields, J.Z., Spokes, E., Bird, E.D. and Yamamura, H.I. (1979), *Life Sci.*, **24**, 809–816.
Bennett, J.P. (1978), *Neurotransmitter Receptor Binding* (Yamamura, H.I., Enna, S.J. and Kuhar, M.J. eds), Raven Press, New York, pp. 56–74.

Berl, S., Nicklas, W.J. and Clarke, D.D. (1970), *J. Neurochem.*, **17**, 1009–1015.

Biscoe, T.J., Davies, J., Dray, A., Evans, R.H., Martin, M.R. and Watkins, J.C. (1978), *Brain Res.*, **148**, 543–548.

Biscoe, T.J., Evans, R.H., Headly, P.M., Martin, M.R. and Watkins, J.C. (1976), *Br. J. Pharmacol.*, **58**, 373–382.

Biziere, K. and Coyle, J.T. (1978a), *J. Neurochem.*, **31**, 513–530.

Biziere, K. and Coyle, J.T. (1978b), *Neurosci. Letts.*, **8**, 303–310.

Biziere, K. and Coyle, J.T. (1979a), *Neuropharmacol.*, **18**, 409–413.

Biziere, K. and Coyle, J.T. (1979b), *J. Neurosci. Res.*, **4**, 383–398.

Biziere, K., Thompson, H. and Coyle, J.T. (1980), *Brain Res.*, **183**, 421–433.

Bradford, H.F. and McIlwain, H. (1966), *J. Neurochem.*, **13**, 1163–1177.

Bradford, H.F. and Richards, C.D. (1976), *Brain Res.*, **111**, 396–398.

Briley, P.A., Kouyoumdjian, J.C., Haidamous, M. and Gonnard, P. (1979), *Europ. J. Pharmacol.*, **54**, 181–184.

Brookes, N. (1979), *Developmental Neurosci.*, **1**, 203–215.

Burt, D.R. (1978), *Neurotransmitter Receptor Binding* (Yamamura, H.I., Enna, S.J. and Kuhar, M.J. eds), Raven Press, New York, pp. 41–55.

Buu, N.T., Puil, E. and van Gelder, N.M. (1976), *Gen. Pharmac.*, **7**, 5–14.

Campochiaro, P. and Coyle, J.T. (1978), *Proc. Natl. Acad. Sci. USA*, **75**, 2025–2029.

Clark, R.B., Gration, K.A.F. and Usherwood, P.N.R. (1979), *Br. J. Pharmacol.*, **66**, 267–273.

Constanti, A. and Nistri, A. (1976), *Br. J. Pharmacol.*, **57**, 359–368.

Constanti, A. and Nistri, A. (1978), *Br. J. Pharmacol.*, **62**, 495–505.

Constanti, A. and Nistri, A. (1979), *Br. J. Pharmacol.*, **65**, 287–301.

Cox, D.W.G. and Bradford, H.F. (1978), *Kainic Acid as a Tool in Neurobiology* (McGeer, E.G., Olney, J.W. and McGeer P.L., eds), Raven Press, New York, pp. 71–93.

Cox, D.W.G., Osborne, R.H. and Watkins, J.C. (1977), *J. Neurochem.*, **29**, 1127–1130.

Coyle, J.T. (1977), *Int. Rev. Neurobiol.*, **20**, 65–103.

Coyle, J.T. (1979), *Biol. Psychiat.*, **14**, 251–276.

Coyle, J.T., Molliver, M.E. and Kuhar, M.J. (1978), *J. Comp. Neurol.*, **180**, 301–323.

Coyle, J.T. and Schwarcz, R. (1976), *Nature*, **263**, 178–180.

Cuatrecasas, P. and Hollenberg, M.D. (1976), *Adv. Protein Chem.*, **30**, 251–451.

Cull-Candy, S.G. (1976), *J. Physiol. (Lond.)*, **255**, 449–464.

Curtis, D.R., Duggan, A.W., Felix, D., Johnston, G.A.R., Tebecis, A.K. and Watkins, J.C. (1972), *Brain Res.*, **41**, 283–301.

Curtis, D.R. and Johnston, G.A.R. (1974), *Ergebn. Physiol.*, **69**, 97–118.

Curtis, D.R., Johnston, G.A.R., Game, S.J.A. and McCulloch, R.M. (1973), *Brain Res.*, **49**, 467–470.

Daoud, A. and Usherwood, P.N.R. (1975), *Comp. Biochem. Physiol.*, **52C**, 51–53.

Davidson, N. (1976), *Neurotransmitter Amino Acids*, Academic Press, New York.

Davies, J. and Dray, A. (1978), *Experientia*, **35**, 353–354.

De Plazas, S.F. and De Robertis, E. (1974), *J. Neurochem.*, **23**, 1115–1120.

De Plazas, S.F. and De Robertis, E. (1976), *J. Neurochem.*, **27**, 889–894.

De Robertis, E. and De Plazas, S.F. (1976), *J. Neurochem.*, **26**, 1237–1243.

DeFrance, J.F., Kitai, S.T. and Shimono, T. (1973), *Exp. Brain Res.*, **17**, 463–476.

DeLean, A., Munson, P.J. and Rodbard, P. (1979), *Mol. Pharmacol.,* **15,** 60–70.

Divak, I., Fonnum, F. and Storm-Mathisen, J. (1977), *Nature,* **266,** 377–378.

Dostrovsky, J.O. and Pomeranz, B. (1977), *Neurosci. Letts.,* **4,** 315–319.

Duggan, W.A. (1974), *Exp. Brain Res.,* **19,** 522–528.

Eusebi, F., Palmieri, P. and Picardo, M. (1978), *Experientia,* **34,** 867–868.

Evans, R.H., Francis, A.A. and Watkins, J.C. (1976), *Experientia,* **33,** 489–491.

Evans, R.H., Franics, A.A. and Watkins, J.C. (1977), *Experientia,* **33,** 246–248.

Evans, R.H., Francis, A.A., Hunt, K., Martin, M.R. and Watkins, J.C. (1978a), *J. Pharm. Pharmacol.,* **30,** 364–367.

Evans, R.H., Francis, A.A. and Watkins, J.C. (1978b), *Brain Res.,* **148,** 536–542.

Faive-Bauman, A., Rossier, J. and Benda, P. (1974), *Brain Res.,* **76,** 371–375.

Ferrendelli, J.A., Chang, M.M. and Kinscherf, D.A. (1974), *J. Neurochem.,* **22,** 535–540.

Florey, E. (1961) *Ann. Rev. Physiol.,* **23,** 501–528.

Florey, E. and Woodcock, B. (1968), *Comp. Biochem. Physiol.,* **26,** 251–261.

Fonnum, F., Karlsen, R.L., Malte-Sorensen, D., Kreda, K.K. and Walaas, J. (1979), *Progress in Brain Res.,* **51,** 375–384.

Foster, A.C. and Roberts, P.J. (1978), *J. Neurochem.,* **31,** 1467–1477.

Freed, W.J. and Michaelis, E.K. (1978), *Pharmacol. Biochem. and Behavior.,* **8,** 509–514.

Gershenfeld, H.M. (1973), *Physiol. Rev.,* **53,** 1–119.

Gration, K.A.F., Clark, R.B. and Usherwood, P.N.R. (1979), *Brain Res.,* **171,** 360–364.

Haldeman, S. and McLennan, H. (1972), *Brain Res.,* **45,** 393–400.

Hall, J.G., Hicks, T.P. and McLennan, H. (1978), *Neurosci. Letts.,* **8,** 171–175.

Hall, J.G., Hicks, T.P., McLennan, H., Richardson, T.L. and Wheal, H.V. (1979), *J. Physiol.,* **286,** 29–39.

Harvey, J.A. and McIlwain, H. (1968), *Biochem. J.,* **108,** 269–274.

Harvey, J.A., Schonfield, C.N., Graham, L.T. and Aprison, M.H. (1975), *J. Neurochem.,* **24,** 445–449.

Hayashi, T. (1954), *Keio. J. Med.,* **3,** 183–192.

Henke, H. and Cuenod, M. (1979), *Neurosci. Letts.,* **11,** 341–345.

Henn, F.A., Goldstein, M. and Hamberger, A. (1974), *Nature,* **249,** 663–664.

Henn, F.A. and Hamberger, A. (1971), *Proc. Natl. Acad. Sci. USA,* **68,** 2686–2690.

Herndon, R.M. and Coyle, J.T. (1977), *Science,* **198,** 71–72.

Hind, J.M. and Kelley, J.S. (1975), *J. Physiol. (Lond),* **2246,** 97–98.

Hosli, Z., Andres, P.F. and Hosli, E. (1976), *Pflugers Arch.,* **363,** 43–48.

Ishida, M. and Shinozaki, H. (1980), *J. Physiol. (Lond.),* in press.

Iversen, L.L. and Kravitz, E.A. (1968), *J. Neurochem.,* **15,** 609–620.

Johnson, J.L. (1972), *Brain Res.,* **37,** 1–19.

Johnson, J.L. (1977), *Life Sci.,* **20,** 1637–1644.

Johnston, G.A.R. (1979), *Glutamic Acid: Advances in Biochemistry and Physiology,* (Filer, L.J., Jr., ed) Raven Press, New York.

Johnston, G.A.R., Allan, R.D., Kennedy, S.M.E. and Twitchin, B. (1978), *GABA Neurotransmitters,* Alfred Benzon Symposium 12, (Krogsgaard-Larsen, P., Scheel-Kruger, J. and Kofod, H., eds.), Munksgaard, pp. 147–156.

Johnston, G.A.R., Kennedy, S.M.E. and Twitchin, B. (1979), *J. Neurochem.*, **32**, 121–127.

Kim, J.S., Hassler, R., Huang, P. and Paik, K.S. (1977), *Brain Res.*, **132**, 370–374.

Kohler, C., Schwarcz, R. and Fuxe, K. (1978), *Neurosci. Letts.*, **10**, 241–246.

Kravitz, E.A., Slater, C.R., Takahashi, K., Bounds, M.D. and Grossfeld, R.M. (1970), *Excitatory Synaptic Mechanisms* (Anderson, P. and Jansen, J.K.S., eds) Universitets Forglaget, Oslo, pp. 85–93.

Krnjevic, K. (1974), *Physiol. Rev.*, **54**, 419–540.

London, E.D. and Coyle, J.T. (1979a), *Eur. J. Pharmacol.* **56**, 287–290.

London, E.D. and Coyle, J.T. (1979b), *Mol. Pharmacol.*, **15**, 492–505.

London, E.D., Klemm, N. and Coyle, J.T. (1980), *Brain Res.*, in press.

Lucas, D.R. and Newhouse, J.P. (1957), *AMA Arch Opthamol.*, **58**, 193–204.

Lund-Karlsen, R. and Fonnum, F. (1978), *Brain Res.*, **151**, 457–467.

Lunt, G.G. (1973), *Comp. Gen. Pharmac.*, **4**, 75–79.

MacDonald, J.F. and Nistri, A. (1977), *Can. J. Physiol. Pharmacol.*, **55** 965–967.

MacDonald, J.F. and Nistri, A. (1978), *J. Physiol.*, **275**, 449–465.

MacDonald, J.F., Nistri, A. and Padjen, A.L. (1977), *Can. J. Physiol. Pharmacol.*, **55**, 1387–1390.

Macdonald, R.L. and Barker, J.L. (1979), *Neurology*, **29**, 432–447.

Marder, E. and Paupardin-Tritsch, D. (1978), *J. Physiol. (Lond.)*, **280**, 213–236.

McBride, W.J., Aprison, M.H. and Kusano, K. (1976a), *J. Neurochem.*, **26**, 867–870.

McBride, W.J., Nadi, N.S., Altman, J. and Aprison, M.H. (1976b), *Neurochem. Res.*, **1**, 141–152.

McBride, W.J., Shank, R.P., Freeman, A.R. and Aprison, M.H. (1974), *Life Sci.*, **19**, 1109–1120.

McBurney, R.N. and Crawford, A.C. (1979), *Fed. Proc.*, **38**, 2080–2083.

McCulloch, R.M., Johnston, G.A.R., Game, C.J.A. and Curtis, D.R. (1974), *Exp. Brain Res.*, **21**, 575–578.

McGeer, E.G. and McGeer, P.L. (1976), *Nature*, **263**, 517–519.

McGeer, E.G., McGeer, P.L. and Singh, K. (1978), *Brain Res.*, **139**, 381–383.

McIlwain, H., Harvey, J.A. and Rodriguez, G. (1969), *J. Neurochem.*, **16**, 363–370.

McLennan, H. (1970), *Synaptic Transmission*, W.B. Saunders, Philadelphia.

McLennan, H. (1975), *Amino Acid Neurotransmitters* (Iversen, L.L., Iversen, S.D. and Snyder, S.H. eds), Plenum Press, New York, pp. 211–234.

McLennan, H. and Lodge, D. (1979), *Brain Res.*, **169**, 83–90.

McLennan, H. and Wheal, H.V. (1978), *Neuroscience Letters*, **8**, 51–54.

Meister, A. (1965), *Biochemistry of the Amino Acids*, Academic Press, New York.

Michaelis, E.K. (1975), *Biochem. Biophys. Res. Commun.*, **65**, 1004–1012.

Michaelis, E.K. (1979), *Biochem. Biophys. Res. Comm.*, **87**, 106–113.

Michaelis, E.K., Michaelis, M.L. and Boyarsky, L.L. (1974), *Biochem. Biophys. Acta.*, **367**, 338–348.

Michaelis, E.K., Mulvaney, M.J. and Freed, W.J. (1978), *Biochem. Pharmacol.*, **27**, 1685–1691.

Miledi, R. (1967), *J. Physiol. (Lond.)*, **92**, 379–406.

Miledi, R. (1972), *J. Physiol. (Lond.)*, **225**, 501–514.

Moore, J.W. and Narahashi, T. (1967), *Fed. Proc.*, **26**, 1655–1663.

Nadler, J.V., Perry, B.W. and Cotman, C.W. (1978), *Nature*, **271**, 676–677.

Nadler, J.V., Vaca, K.W., White, W.F., Lynch, G.S. and Cotman, C.W. (1976), *Nature*, **260**, 538–540.

Nadler, J.V., White, W.F., Vaca, K.W., Perry, B.W. and Cotman, C.W. (1978), *J. Neurochem.*, **31**, 147–155.

Neal, M.J. (1976), *Gen. Pharmacol.*, **7**, 321–332.

Okamoto, K. and Quastel, J.H. (1972), *Biochem. J.*, **128**, 1117–1124.

Olney, J.W. (1969), *Science*, **164**, 719–721.

Olney, J.W. (1971), *J. Neuropathol. Exp. Neurol.*, **30**, 75–90.

Olney, J.W. and de Gubareff, T. (1978a), *Brain Res.*, **140**, 340–343.

Olney, J.W. and de Gubareff, T. (1978b), *Nature*, **271**, 557–559.

Olney, J.W., de Gubareff, T. and Labuyeve, J. (1979), *Life Sci.*, **6**, 537–540.

Olney, J.W., Ho., O.L. and Rhee, V. (1971), *Exp. Brain Res.*, **14**, 61–76.

Perry, T.L., Currier, R.D., Hansen, S. and MacLean, J. (1977), *Neurology*, **27**, 257–261.

Phillis, J.W. (1966), *The Pharmacology of Synapses*, Pergamon Press, New York.

Polc, P. and Haefely, W. (1977), *Naunyn-Schmiedeberg's Arch. Pharmacol.*, **300**, 199–203.

Ransom, B.R., Bullock, P.N. and Nelson, P.G. (1977), *J. Neurophysiol.*, **40**, 1163–1177.

Richards, C.D. and Smaje, J.C. (1976), *Br. J. Pharmacol.*, **58**, 347–357.

Roberts, P.J. (1974), *Nature*, **252**, 399–401.

Schmidt, M.J., Ryan, J.J. and Molloy, B.B. (1976), *Brain Res.*, **112**, 113–126.

Schmidt, M.J., Thornberry, J.F. and Molloy, B.B. (1977), *Brain Res.*, **121**, 182–189.

Schwarcz, R. and Coyle, J.T. (1977), *Invest. Opthamol.*, **16**, 141–149.

Schwarcz, R. and Fuxe, K. (1979), *Life Sci.*, **24**, 1471–1480.

Schwarcz, R., Hokfelt, T., Fuxe, K., Jonsson, G., Goldstein, M. and Terenius, L. (1980), *Exp. Brain Res.*, **37**, 199–216.

Schwarcz, R., Scholz, D. and Coyle, J.T. (1978), *Neuropharmacol.*, **17**, 145–151.

Segal, M. (1977), *Brain Res.*, **119**, 476–479.

Shank, R.P. and Freeman, A.R. (1975), *J. Neurobiol.*, **6**, 289–303.

Shank, R.P. and Freeman, A.R. (1976), *J. Neurobiol.*, **7**, 23–36.

Shank, R.P., Wang, M.B. and Freeman, A.R. (1977), *Brain Res.*, **126**, 176–180.

Shimizu, H., Ichishita, H. and Odagiri, H. (1974), *J. Biol. Chem.*, **249**, 5955–5962.

Shimizu, H., Ichishita, H. and Umeda, I. (1975), *Mol. Pharmacol.*, **11**, 866–873.

Shinozaki, H. and Ishida, M. (1976), *Brain Res.*, **109**, 435–439.

Shinozaki, H. and Ishida, M. (1979), *Brain Res.*, **161**, 493–501.

Shinozaki, H. and Konishi, S. (1970), *Brain Res.*, **24**, 368–371.

Shinozaki, H. and Shibuya, I. (1974), *Neuropharmacology*, **13**, 1057–1065.

Shinozaki, H. and Shibuya, I. (1976), *Neuropharmacology*, **15**, 145–147.

Simon, J.R., Contrera, J.F. and Kuhar, M.J. (1976), *J. Neurochem.*, **26**, 141–147.

Snyder, S.H. and Bennett, J.P. (1976), *Ann. Rev. Physiol.*, **38**, 153–175.

Spencer, H.J. (1976), *Brain Res.*, **102**, 91–101.

Stone, T.W. (1979), *Br. J. Pharmacol.*, **66**, 291–296.

Storm-Mathisen, J. and Opsahl, M.W. (1978), *Neurosci. Letts.*, **9**, 65–70.

Takemoto, T. (1978), *Kainic Acid as a Tool in Neurobiology* (McGeer, E.G., Olney, J.W. and McGeer, P.L., eds), Raven Press, New York, pp. 1–15.

Takeuchi, A. and Onodera, K. (1975), *Neuropharmacology*, **14**, 619–625.

Thieffry, M. and Bruner, J. (1978), *Brain Res.*, **156**, 402–406.

Valcana, T., Hudson, D. and Timiras, P.S. (1972), *J. Neurochem.*, **19**, 2229–2232.

Van Harreveld, A. and Fifkova, E. (1971), *Exp. Mol. Pathol.*, **15**, 61–81.

Vincent, S.R. and McGeer, E.G. (1979), *Life Sci.*, **24**, 265–270.

Walker, R.J. (1976), *Comp. Biochem. Physiol.*, **55C**, 61–67.

Watkins, J.C. (1978), *Kainic Acid as a Tool in Neurobiology* (McGeer, E.G., Olney, J.W., and McGeer, P.L., eds), Raven Press, New York, pp. 37–69.

Watkins, J.C., Curtis, D.R. and Brand, S.J. (1977), *J. Pharm. Pharmacol.*, **29**, 234.

Wenthold, R.J. (1978), *Brain Res.*, **143**, 544–548.

Wenthold, R.J. and Gulley, R.L. (1978), *Brain Res.*, **158**, 295–302.

Wheal, H.V. and Kerkut, G.A. (1976), *Comp. Biochem. Physiol.*, **53C**, 51–55.

White, W.F., Nadler, J.V., Hamberger, A., Cotman, C.W. and Cummins, J.T. (1977), *Nature*, **270**, 356–357.

Wu, S.M. and Dowling, J.E. (1978), *Proc. Natl. Acad. Sci. USA*, **75**, 5205–5209.

Yamamoto, C. and Matsui, S. (1976), *J. Neurochem.*, **26**, 487–491.

Yarowsky, P.J. and Carpenter, D.O. (1976), *Science*, **192**, 807–809.

Yokoi, I., Takeuchi, H., Sakai, A. and Mori, A. (1976), *Experientia*, **33**, 363–366.

Young, A.B., Oster-Granite, M.L., Herndon, R.M. and Snyder, S.H. (1974), *Brain Res.*, **73**, 1–13.

Zaczek, R., Hedreen, J. and Coyle, J.T. (1979), *Exp. Neurol.*, **65**, 145–156.

Zaczek, R., Nelson, M.F. and Coyle, J.T. (1978), *Eur. J. Pharmacol.*, **52**, 323–327.

Zieglgansberger, W. and Puil, E.A. (1973), *Exp. Brain Res.*, **17**, 35–49.

2 Glycine, GABA and Benzodiazepine Receptors

S.J. ENNA and JON F. DeFRANCE

Acknowledgements
Preparation of this chapter was facilitated by USPHS grants MH-31114, NS-13803, a Research Career Development award NS-00335 (S.J.E.) and a grant from the Scottish Rite Schizophrenia Research Program. We thank Ms. Jill McCoig for her excellent secretarial assistance.

Neurotransmitter Receptors Part 1
(*Receptors and Recognition*, Series B, Volume 9)
Edited by S.J. Enna and H.I. Yamamura
Published in 1980 by Chapman and Hall, 11 New Fetter Lane,
London EC4P 4EE
© Chapman and Hall

2.1 INTRODUCTION

While a neurotransmitter function for amino acids in the mammalian central nervous system was suspected for a number of years, it was not until the late 1950s, with the development of intracellular recording techniques, that physiologists were able to demonstrate that these simple substances could directly alter the electrical potential of individual neurons. As a result of these studies, amino acid neurotransmitter candidates have been classified as either inhibitory or excitatory, depending upon the electrophysiological response to the agent (Curtis *et al.*, 1959, 1960; Davidson, 1976; Enna, 1979a). To date, twelve amino acids have been tentatively identified as inhibitory neurotransmitters while four have properties characteristic of an excitatory transmitter agent (Curtis and Johnston, 1974a). Of the twelve potential inhibitory amino acids, two, γ-aminobutyric acid (GABA) and glycine, have been extensively studied because there are relatively specific pharmacological antagonists for these substances. Thus, the convulsant bicuculline is much more potent in inhibiting GABA than glycine responses, whereas the convulsant strychnine antagonizes the effects of glycine but is relatively ineffective on GABA (Phillis et al., 1968; Curtis and Tebēcis, 1972). Accordingly, inhibitory amino acids are often classified as glycine-like or GABA-like to indicate which convulsant is more potent in blocking the action of the agent.

The present chapter describes the physiological, biochemical and pharmacological properties of synaptic receptor sites for GABA and glycine. In addition, some properties of the receptor for benzodiazepines, widely used anxiolytic agents, will also be briefly discussed since recent experimental evidence suggests that the receptor for these drugs may be linked to inhibitory amino acid receptor sites, particularly GABA receptors.

2.2 GENERAL BIOCHEMICAL CONSIDERATIONS

2.2.1 Glycine

Probably the first solid biochemical evidence to indicate a neurotransmitter role for glycine was accumulated during the fruitful collaboration of Werman, Aprison and their colleagues (Aprison and Werman, 1965; Davidoff *et al.*, 1967a, b; Graham *et al.*, 1967). These workers demonstrated a distinct regional distribution for glycine within the mammalian spinal cord, with levels being significantly higher in the ventral than in the dorsal gray, whereas very little of the amino acid was found in either the ventral or dorsal white matter. These investigators noted that this distribution would be expected of the natural inhibitory neurotransmitter, since the cell bodies and axons of the inhibitory neurons should be contained predominantly in gray matter. Further evidence was provided by the finding that the content of glycine, but not other amino acids, was significantly reduced in the ventral gray of cats whose spinal cords had been subjected to prolonged anoxia, a condition which was known to lead to a selective loss of spinal interneurons. In addition, they were able to demonstrate that the decrease in glycine levels correlated in a positive manner with the loss of spinal neurons indicating that this amino acid was highly concentrated in these nerve cells. Thus, in the spinal cord at least, the concentration of glycine is compatible with a neurotransmitter function.

Like other putative neurotransmitter substances, glycine is accumulated by a high-affinity uptake system in central nervous tissue, with uptake being most enriched in spinal cord and brain stem areas (Neal and Pickles, 1969; Johnston and Iversen, 1971; Logan and Snyder, 1972). Autoradiographic studies have indicated that the nerve terminal is the major site of glycine accumulation in spinal cord (Matus and Dennison, 1971). Using spinal cord synaptosomes, Iversen and Bloom (1972) have reported that approximately 30 per cent of the total synaptosomal population accumulates ^{3}H-glycine, suggesting that a significant number of spinal cord neurons utilize glycine as a transmitter.

In addition to having a specific neuronal localization and high-affinity transport system, glycine is released from the dorsal roots of the hemisectioned toad spinal cord in a frequency-dependent fashion following electrical stimulation (Aprison, 1970). Furthermore, radiolabeled glycine is released from the isolated toad and frog hemicord after electrical stimulation of the rostral cord and, *in vitro*, studies have demonstrated a calcium-dependent release of glycine from both spinal cord slices and synaptosomal fractions (Hopkins and Neal, 1970; Hammerstad *et al.*, 1971; Roberts and Mitchell, 1972; Osborne *et al.*, 1973).

With regard to metabolism, three major pathways for glycine synthesis have been described in nervous tissue (Bridgers, 1965; Johnston *et al.*, 1970; Uhr and Sneddon, 1972). Based on current evidence, the major pathway for glycine synthesis in the central nervous system appears to be from glucose and serine by way of a nonphosphorylated pathway. Evidence also indicates that D-glycerate dehydrogenase, which converts D-glycerate to hydroxypyruvate, and serine hydroxymethyltransferase, which catalyses the conversion of serine to glycine, are the rate-limiting enzymes for the biosynthesis of glycine in nervous tissue (Roberts and Hammerschlag, 1976). With regard to catabolism, glycine is incorporated into proteins or glutathione in nervous tissue (Douglas and Martensen, 1965; Mase *et al.*,

1962; Globus *et al.*, 1968) or it can be converted back to serine or glyoxylate by way of serine hydroxymethyltransferase or transamination, respectively (Roberts and Hammerschlag, 1976).

Thus, glycine is present in specific neuronal elements, particularly in the spinal cord and brain stem regions and this amino acid can be synthesized, catabolized, transported and released from these neurons. This evidence is consistent with the notion that glycine serves a neurotransmitter function in mammalian central nervous tissue.

2.2.2 GABA

Of all the amino acid neurotransmitter candidates, GABA has probably been the most thoroughly investigated. The biochemical evidence supporting a neurotransmitter function for GABA is substantial and has been the subject of a number of reviews (Curtis and Johnston, 1974a; DeFeudis, 1975; Davidson, 1976; Fonnum, 1978; Krogsgaard-Larsen *et al.*, 1979). Briefly, like other neurotransmitter candidates, there is a heterogenous distribution of GABA and the enzymes involved in its synthesis and degradation (Fahn, 1976). In addition, GABA is highly concentrated in a distinct synaptosomal population (Kuhar *et al.*, 1970, 1971), there is a high-affinity transport for the amino acid in brain (Iversen and Neal, 1968; Roberts and Kuriyama, 1968), and a calcium-dependent GABA release from brain tissue has been reported (Redburn *et al.*, 1978). Finally, the GABA-containing neurons in the central nervous system have been identified and their anatomical distribution catalogued using both immunocytochemical and autoradiographic techniques (Iversen and Bloom, 1972; McLaughlin *et al.*, 1974). GABA is synthesized in neurons primarily from glutamic acid, a reaction which is catalysed by the enzyme glutamic acid decarboxylase (Roberts and Frankel, 1950) and it is catabolized by the enzyme GABA-α-ketoglutarate transaminase (GABA-T) to succinic semialdehyde. Relatively specific inhibitors of high-affinity GABA transport, metabolism, and direct-acting receptor agonists and antagonists have been developed, which have helped to define the pharmacological characteristics of this system (Enna and Maggi, 1979).

2.3 RECEPTOR CHARACTERISTICS

2.3.1 Ionic mechanisms of receptor action

Inhibitory postsynaptic potentials (IPSPs) were first recorded, intra-cellularly, in spinal neurons (Brock *et al.*, 1952). These postsynaptic hyperpolarizations serve to suppress cellular discharge, providing the basis for 'direct inhibition' (Lloyd, 1941). Since these early explorations, IPSPs have been recorded throughout the nervous system. These synaptic potentials are the primary way in which the nervous system organizes excitatory–inhibitory sequences.

Glycine and GABA are two chemical messengers which produce 'fast' IPSPs[1] in CNS neurons. The character of the conductance changes giving rise to 'fast' IPSPs has been determined by varying the concentrations of different ions and recording the changes in the IPSP amplitude and duration (Coombs *et al.*, 1955; Araki *et al.*, 1961; Eccles *et al.*, 1964a, b). Apparently, all 'fast' IPSPs are similar with regard to their mechanism of generation such that the hyperpolarization results from a flux of ionic current out of the subsynaptic portion of the cell. The current flow results from specific conductance changes to Cl^- and perhaps, K^+ (Coombs *et al.*, 1955). These events follow receptor activation. Thus, GABA or glycine binds to the receptor which, in some way, facilitates the entry of Cl^- to the cell and, possibly, the exit of K^+, resulting in an outward flow of current. The consequence of this current flow is hyperpolarization of the neuron, since the membrane potential moves away from the Cl^- equilibrium potential towards the IPSP equilibrium potential. The equilbrium potential is that transmembrane potential at which there is no net flux of an ion(s) across the membrane. The observation that the Cl^- and IPSP equilibrium potentials are different led to the suggestion that K^+ may also be involved. However, a movement of K^+ need not be postulated if there exists a Cl^- pump that normally maintains the internal concentrations of Cl^- below the concentration that would exist as a result of passive diffusion alone (Eccles *et al.*, 1964a, b). In any event, the transient increase in Cl^- conductance appears to be the critical event for the generation of 'fast' IPSPs.

Glycine appears to be one of the primary messengers mediating 'fast' IPSPs in the spinal cord (Werman *et al.*, 1967, 1968; Curtis *et al.*, 1968a) and medullary reticular formation (Hosli and Tebēcis, 1970; Haas and Hosli, 1973). The nature of this effect has been clarified by studies with spinal motoneurons. Thus, glycine induces a transient hyperpolarization in these neurons (Curtis *et al.*, 1968b; ten Bruggencate and Engberg, 1968; Werman *et al.*, 1968) that, like the 'fast' IPSP, is accompanied by an increase in the conductance of small ions (Curtis *et al.*, 1968b; Werman *et al.*, 1968). Injections of Cl^- converts both the glycine hyperpolarization and IPSP evoked by electrical stimulation to a depolarization. Also, the equilibrium potential for the glycine-mediated hyperpolarization and IPSP are similar (Werman and Aprison, 1968). Werman *et al.* (1968) found that this increase in membrane conductance averages around 50 per cent, whereas the decrease in membrane resistance was approximately 35 per cent. This

---

[1]Please see review by Weight (1974) for differences between 'fast' and 'slow' IPSPs.

evidence supports the notion that glycine receptor activation preferentially affects Cl⁻ conductance. There seems to be no desensitization of the receptor associated with this glycine effect (Werman *et al.*, 1968; Krnjevic *et al.*, 1977a) since the suppressive action is maintained as long as glycine is applied.

In addition to suppressing cellular action potentials, glycine can also affect the amplitude of synaptic potentials (Curtis *et al.*, 1968a; Werman *et al.*, 1968) since both IPSPs and EPSPs are diminished in strength by a shunting effect of the increase in membrane conductance.

It is noteworthy that glycine is ineffective when injected intracellularly (Werman *et al.*, 1968), which implies that the glycine-mediated IPSP involves receptor activation. From his studies, Werman (1975) has suggested that glycine receptors require the attachment of at least two glycine molecules.

Further evidence that the glycine effect is a receptor-mediated phenomenon was provided by studying the interaction of the glycine-induced hyperpolarization with various pharmacological agents. Curtis *et al.* (1967) discovered that the glycine hyperpolarization of motor neurons was antagonized by strychnine and strychnine-like compounds (e.g. thebaine and bruceine). There is some controversy, however, as to the specificity of the strychnine antagonism since, as pointed out by Phillis and York (1967), strychnine may also antagonize monoamine-induced depression in the cerebral cortex. Strychnine has also been reported to antagonize the effects of acetylcholine and histamine (Phillis and York, 1968a, b). Hence, a strychnine effect should not be taken as the sole criterion for the specificity of glycine's action at a receptor. Other substances which have been reported to antagonize the suppressive effect of glycine are morphine (Curtis and Duggan, 1969) and some indole alkaloids (Curtis and Johnston, 1974b; Johnston, 1976a).

In the spinal cord, glycine is an effector on dendritic and somatic membranes, whereas in this region, GABA appears to have both a significant pre- and postsynaptic action. The receptor mechanisms for the postsynaptic action of GABA in the brain and spinal cord is similar to that of glycine. Receptor activation leads to an increase in Cl⁻ conductance with a resultant hyperpolarization (Curtis *et al.*, 1968b; Werman *et al.*, 1968; Krnjevic *et al.*, 1977b). The postsynaptic effect of GABA may be characterized as being potent, with a rapid onset and a short latency to maximal effect (Krnjevic and Phillis, 1963).

In a detailed study of the GABA effect in cultured spinal neurons, Ransom and Barker (1976) found that the GABA induced hyperpolarization decays in such a way as to suggest two phases of relaxation of the conductance channels. There seems to be an early phase which is characterized by a fall in conductance, and a later phase where the decline proceeds more slowly. These observations suggest that there may exist more than one type of GABA receptor. With respect to glycine, GABA-induced conductance changes return more slowly. As a possible consequence of this action, GABA-mediated IPSPs may be longer in duration than those induced by glycine.

Like glycine, GABA has an effect on the amplitude of synaptic potentials, with the GABA-mediated hyperpolarizations reducing the influence of EPSPs and IPSPs through a shunting effect (Curtis *et al.*, 1968b). However, unlike the postsynaptic action of glycine, the effects of GABA appear to be subject to receptor desensitization (Curtis *et al.*, 1959; Krnjevic *et al.*, 1977b; Krnjevic and Phillis, 1963). 'Desensitization' is a diminution of an effect as a result of repeated or prolonged application of a substance. This phenomenon correlates with a decrease in the GABA-induced conductance change (Dreifuss *et al.*, 1969; Krnjevic *et al.*, 1977b), and it has been proposed that the desensitization is due to receptor inactivation (Katz and Thesleff, 1957).

GABA is clearly different from glycine with respect to pharmacological antagonism. Whereas strychnine blocks glycine suppression, it has no influence on GABA-mediated effects. On the other hand, bicuculline (and closely related compounds) effectively antagonize the GABA, but not glycine-induced suppression (e.g. Krnjevic *et al.*, 1977a). Similarly, picrotoxin blocks the action of GABA, but not glycine.

With regard to GABA receptors mediating presynaptic inhibition, this type of response was first described in spinal afferent fibers by Frank and Fuortes (1957) and later by Eccles *et al.* (1962, 1963). The anatomical basis for this type of inhibition are axo-axonic synapses made by interneurons upon afferent fibers. Therefore, a volley of impulses will excite target projection neurons, while at the same time activating interneurons. The interneurons in turn project to, and stimulate, the terminals of afferent fibers impinging upon the projection cells. Since these interneurons are presumed to depolarize (excite) the afferent fibers in the terminal areas (Eccles, 1964) it has been referred to as primary afferent depolarization (PAD). Such a depolarization would reduce the amplitude of the next action potential and, since the amount of transmitter released is proportional to the amplitude of the potential change in the terminal area, the amount of transmitter released from the afferent fibers is reduced. This series of events is referred to as presynaptic, indirect, or remote (Frank, 1959) inhibition.

It was suggested by Eccles *et al.* (1963) that the chemical messenger of the interneuron was GABA, since this form of inhibition was strychnine resistant, but picrotoxin sensitive. Subsequently, other pharmacological studies have supported the notion that GABA is involved in PAD, since bicuculline has also been shown to antagonize this effect (Barker and Nicoll, 1972; Barker *et al.*, 1975; Davidoff, 1977). Consistent with these findings, evidence for the participation of Cl^- conductance changes has been presented (Deschenes *et al.*, 1976; Otsuka and Konishi, 1976). Glycine has been shown to have no consistent effect on afferent terminal excitability (Curtis *et al.*, 1967).

The apparent involvement of Cl^- in PAD raises the interesting question as to how an increase in Cl^- conductance can depolarize the terminal area. In an attempt to address this issue, de Groat (1972) and Nishi *et al.* (1974) reported that peripheral nerve cells have a high internal Cl^- concentration, maintained by an inwardly directed Cl^- pump. If such a pump were able to keep intracellular Cl^- higher than equilibrium levels, then a Cl^- conductance increase would cause a depolarizing response since the flow of this ion would be outward rather than inward. Furthermore, there also appears to be a desensitization to this GABA effect (Dreifuss *et al.*, 1969; Adams and Brown, 1973). This interpretation of the data is attractive in that it preserves the integrity of the notion that GABA receptors regulate Cl^- channels. However, other interpretations are possible.

Barron and Matthews (1938) demonstrated that the discharge of afferent fibers can result in the accumulation of extracellular K^+, which, rather than intracellular Cl^-, could be the ionic basis for PAD. This suggestion has been supported by a number of studies (e.g. Krnjevic and Morris, 1974, 1975; Lothman and Somjen, 1975). The effects of extracellular K^+ on the release of neurotransmitters are well documented (Weight and Frulkar, 1979). This theory suggests that extracellular K^+ causes a partial depolarization of the presynaptic elements which causes a reduction in the amplitude of the next action potential, which in turn would lead to a reduction of transmitter release. Thus, with the K^+ theory, there is no need for a presynaptic receptor for GABA. Perhaps both ionic mechanisms are operative in the spinal cord.

A complicating factor of GABA receptor physiology is that this amino acid has effects on cell populations having no apparent GABAergic input. It is known that GABA depolarizes sensory ganglion cells, which are without GABA synapses (de Groat, 1972; Obata, 1972; Deschenes *et al.*, 1976). Furthermore, in the initial description of the effect of GABA on cortical cells, Krnjevic and Schwartz (1966, 1967) pointed out that GABA depolarizes glial cells, but without a significant conductance change. Similarly, GABA depolarizes sympathetic ganglionic cells (Adams and Brown, 1975; Bowery and Brown, 1974). However, the ganglionic depolarization is reported to be accompanied by a conductance change to Cl^- (Adams and Brown, 1973). With respect to ganglionic cell populations, the effects exhibit desensitization. Krnjevic *et al.* (1977b) have further shown that although the conductance increase to GABA is blocked by bicuculline, this alkaloid does not block the depolarizing effect. An explanation for these findings might be the electrogenic uptake of GABA by cortical cells (Henn and Hamburger, 1971; Schon *et al.*, 1975). This amino acid transport appears to be dependent upon a sodium influx (Schultz and Curran, 1970; Christensen, 1973), but during the uptake of neutral amino acids there is an associated depolarization which would not be blocked by bicuculline (Rose and Schultz, 1970; Oomura *et al.*, 1974; Laris *et al.*, 1976). Such an active uptake of GABA could also account for the GABA receptor 'desensitization' (Krnjevic *et al.*, 1977b).

On the other hand, if these cells have high internal levels of Cl⁻, a depolarization would result simply from the reverse of the electrochemical gradient during the conductance change (Adams and Brown, 1973), as has been proposed for PAD in the spinal cord.

Another contrast between GABA and glycine receptors comes from the studies of the mechanism of action of the benzodiazepines. There is considerable evidence that benzodiazepines exert their effect by way of GABA receptor mechanisms. Costa *et al.* (1975) and Haefely *et al.*, (1975) proposed that the benzodiazepines facilitate transmission at GABAergic synapses. Furthermore, while MacDonald and Barker (1978) found that the benzodiazepines enhance GABA-mediated postsynaptic inhibition in the spinal cord using small ejection currents, higher currents antagonized the GABA effect. While the exact relationship between benzodiazepines and GABA receptors still remains to be clarified, the many effects of the benzodiazepines have lead Curtis *et al.* (1976b) to suggest that there may be more than a single type of GABA receptor. Benzodiazepines appear to have no effect on glycine-mediated responses (Curtis *et al.*, 1968b).

2.3.2 Biochemical characteristics of glycine receptors

The development of a ligand binding assay to study the glycine receptor (Young and Snyder, 1973) facilitated the biochemical definition of this site. Using rat central nervous system subcellular fractions, these investigators demonstrated that the glycine receptor antagonist, ³H-strychnine, binds in a saturable and specific fashion with an affinity constant of approximately 30 nM. That this binding represents attachment to the glycine receptor was indicated by the fact that the potency of various amino acids to displace ³H-strychnine paralleled their ability to mimic the neurophysiological actions of glycine. In this assay, both glycine and β-alanine, a glycine-like inhibitory substance, caused a half-maximal displacement of ³H-strychnine binding at concentrations of about 10 μM. In addition, the convulsant potencies of a number of strychnine analogs paralleled their ability to displace ³H-strychnine from crude synaptic membranes of rat spinal cord and medulla (Mackerer, 1977). Further evidence that specific ³H-strychnine binding represents attachment to the glycine receptor was provided by the finding that it is most enriched in subcellular fractions known to contain the highest concentration of synaptic membranes, and the central nervous system regional distribution of the binding is similar to the regional distribution of electrophysiological sensitivity to glycine and to high-affinity glycine uptake (Young and Snyder, 1973). Thus, in rat central nervous tissue, binding was greatest in the spinal cord and medulla followed by midbrain, hypothalamus and thalamus. In contrast, cerebellum, hippocampus, corpus striatum and cerebral cortex display negligible binding activity.

Using the ^{3}H-strychnine binding assay, glycine receptors have been identified in rat, monkey, pigeon and frog central nervous system tissues (Young and Snyder, 1973; LeFort *et al.*, 1978; Muller and Snyder, 1978a). In all species studied, the pharmacological and biochemical characteristics of the receptor appear to be similar. However, the regional distribution of ^{3}H-strychnine binding differs in the frog, as compared to the other species, in that the frog cerebral cortex binds a significant amount of the ligand suggesting that synaptic glycine receptors may be present in the higher brain centers of this species.

Equilibrium binding saturation studies indicate that ^{3}H-strychnine labels a single population of sites and that glycine interacts with this site in a co-operative fashion, with a Hill coefficient for glycine displacement of ^{3}H-strychnine of 1.7 (Young and Snyder, 1974a). Furthermore, protein-modifying reagents such as diazonium tetrazole and acetic anhydride and certain inorganic ions can differentially affect the ability of strychnine and glycine to inhibit ^{3}H-strychnine binding (Young and Snyder, 1974a; Muller and Snyder, 1978b). These data, taken together, indicate that glycine and strychnine attach to distinct, but interacting sites (Young and Snyder, 1974a). The possible identity of the two sites on the glycine receptor was revealed by other experiments indicating that inorganic anions are capable of inhibiting ^{3}H-strychnine binding and that their relative potencies in this regard parallel their ability to reverse neuronal inhibitory postsynaptic potentials (Young and Snyder, 1974b). Thus anions capable of mimicking Cl^- electrophysiologically are capable of inhibiting ^{3}H-strychnine binding; whereas anions, which because of their relatively large hydration radius are incapable of crossing the glycine-activated Cl^- channel, are also incapable of inhibiting ^{3}H-strychnine binding. These findings suggest that ^{3}H-strychnine interacts with, or perhaps attaches, to, the ionophore portion of the glycine receptor, while glycine itself attaches to the recognition site of the receptor. This notion of a co-operative interaction between glycine and strychnine has some physiological precedent in that neurophysiological studies have indicated that GABA interacts in a co-operative fashion with the antagonist picrotoxin (Brooks and Werman, 1973).

The results of these studies are therefore in accord with the notion that glycine attaches to the recognition site on the postsynaptic receptor, activating a change in ionic conductance at a portion of the receptor which is distinct from, but intimately related to, the recognition site. Strychnine, on the other hand, appears not to bind to the recognition site, but rather to some portion of the receptor, possibly the ionophore, which is influenced by the attachment of glycine. This being the case, there are at least two ways in which glycine receptors can be blocked; by antagonists which will bind to the recognition site and by antagonists which will bind to the strychnine site. If a single ion channel can be activated by a number of different receptor agonists acting at different recognition sites, this finding may explain why strychnine is capable of reversing the action of a number of amino acids, such as β-alanine and taurine (Curtis *et al.*, 1968a).

With regard to other biochemical aspects of the glycine receptor, unlike the catecholamines and glutamic acid, no glycine-stimulated cyclic nucleotide system has yet been found in nerve tissue. However, glycine has been reported to inhibit dopamine release in the caudate nucleus of the cat (Cheramy *et al.*, 1978a). In this study, superfusion of the cat substantia nigra with glycine (10–5 M), causes a decrease in the spontaneous release of ^{3}H-dopamine in the ipsilateral caudate nucleus. This glycine effect is strychnine-sensitive and is in accord with neurophysiological studies indicating that glycine blocks nerve firing in the pars compacta and pars reticulata of the substantia nigra (Dray and Gonye, 1975; Dray *et al.*, 1976; Crossman *et al.*, 1973). These reports suggest that glycine may play a neurotransmitter role in the substantia nigra and that it may be the transmitter mediating the effect of nigral interneurons (Cheramy *et al.*, 1978a). Thus, while binding and electrophysiological studies have indicated that glycine receptors are most abundant in the spinal cord and brain stem, it is likely that glycine may also play an important, though limited, role as a neurotransmitter in other brain regions.

Little work has been done in developing pharmacological agonists or antagonists for the glycine receptor. This paucity of pharmacological tools has hindered more complete investigations into the molecular, and behavioral, consequences of glycine receptor activation or inhibition. From a chemical standpoint, the major difficulty in developing glycine receptor-specific agents is the simple nature of the molecule, since the structure of glycine leaves little room for chemical manipulation. Nevertheless, the development, or discovery of glycine receptor agonists or antagonists would be a boon to the further biochemical and physiological characterization of this site.

2.3.3 Biochemical characteristics of GABA receptors

Early studies on GABA binding to brain tissue focused on a sodium-dependent binding system (Varon *et al.*, 1965; Kuriyama *et al.*,

1968; Roberts and Kuriyama, 1968; Gottesfeld and Elliott, 1971; DeFeudis, 1973). However, the development of ^{3}H-GABA having a greater specific activity led to the discovery of a higher affinity, sodium-independent binding site possessing the pharmacological characteristics of the synaptic receptor site for this amino acid (Zukin *et al.*, 1974; Enna and Snyder, 1975). Using this ligand, it was found that the sodium-dependent binding probably represents attachment to the sodium-dependent GABA transport system on neurons and glia, whereas the sodium-independent site has the characteristics expected of the synaptic receptor site (Enna and Snyder, 1975; Greenlee *et al.*, 1978a; Lester and Peck, 1979; Winkler *et al.*, 1979). More recently, the pharmacological and biochemical characteristics of the GABA receptor in mammalian brain have been studied using the agonist ^{3}H-muscimol (Beaumont *et al.*, 1978; Leach and Wilson, 1978; Snodgrass, 1978), and the antagonists ^{3}H-bicuculline (Mohler and Okada, 1977a, 1978) and ^{3}H-dihydropicrotoxinin (Ticku *et al.*, 1978; Ticku and Olsen, 1978) for labeling this site. Using these different ligands, it appears that both GABA and muscimol bind to the same population of receptors (Enna *et al.*, 1978), but the binding of bicuculline, while apparently to the GABA receptor recognition site, has pharmacological and brain distribution characteristics suggesting that there may be conformational differences between the agonist and antagonist binding sites (Mohler and Okada, 1978). In contrast, ^{3}H-dihydropicrotoxinin does not appear to label the receptor recognition site since neither GABA receptor agonists nor bicuculline are very potent in displacing this radioligand. Rather, the pharmacological characteristics of ^{3}H-dihydropicrotoxinin binding indicate that it may attach to the ionophore portion of the GABA receptor (Olsen *et al.*, 1978).

Using ^{3}H-GABA, sodium-independent GABA receptors have been identified in the brain, spinal cord and retina of various vertebrate species including man (Enna *et al.*, 1975, 1976, 1977a; Enna and Snyder, 1975, 1976, 1977a; Mann and Enna, 1979). Furthermore, by studying the influence of various enzymes, detergents and inorganic ions on sodium-independent ^{3}H-GABA binding to rat brain membranes it was found that chaotropic agents, such as the ammonium salts of thiocyanate, iodide and nitrate, increase the potency of bicuculline to displace ^{3}H-GABA from the receptor, but do not alter the potency of agonists as binding site inhibitors, further suggesting some differences between the properties of the agonist and antagonist binding sites (Enna and Snyder, 1977b). It was also found that preincubating brain membranes with the nonionic detergent Triton X-100 enhances the apparent affinity of the receptor ten-fold for agonists, but has no effect on antagonists. Subsequent investigations have indicated that rigorous washing of the membranes, like treatment with Triton, removes an 'endogenous inhibitor(s)' of ^{3}H-GABA receptor binding (Wong and and Horng, 1977; Greenlee, *et al.*, 1978b; Johnston and

Kennedy, 1978; Toffano *et al.*, 1978). This 'endogenous inhibitor(s)' or 'modulator(s)' may be a protein or a phospholipid, or both, and it appears that its presence at or near the GABA receptor can allosterically alter the conformational structure of the receptor recognition site such that removal of this substance(s) results in an increased affinity of the receptor for GABA, which in turn leads to an enhancement of GABAergic transmission. This novel hypothesis has profound implications from both a molecular and pharmacological standpoint since it suggests a new and rapid acting mechanism for regulating receptor sensitivity and it implies that, if such a mechanism exists, it may be manipulated pharmacologically for therapeutic gain. Indeed, studies have shown that the benzodiazepines may enhance GABAergic transmission by displacing this GABA receptor 'modulator' substance(s) (see below).

With regard to the development and localization of GABA receptors, binding studies in rat brain have indicated that the receptor is present at birth and that the number of receptors begins to increase dramatically at 8 days of age, reaching adult levels by one month after birth (Coyle and Enna, 1976). The regional distribution of GABA receptor binding is similar in rat and human brain, being highest in the cerebellum and cerebral cortex, with intermediate to low values found in the corpus striatum, midbrain, brain stem and spinal cord (Enna and Snyder, 1975; Enna *et al.*, 1977a).

Within the cerebellum, granule cell lesion experiments have indicated that up to 60 per cent of the GABA receptors are localized to this cell type (Simantov *et al.*, 1976). In contrast, using an autoradiographic technique with ^{3}H-muscimol, it has been reported that the highest binding occurs on Purkinje cells (Chan-Palay, 1978). However, there is some question about the pharmacological specificity of the ^{3}H-muscimol binding observed in this study, and a more recent autoradiographic investigation, using an *in vitro* labeling technique, has found that the greatest accumulation of ^{3}H-muscimol is, in fact, on granule cells (Palacios *et al.*, 1979). The precise cellular localization of GABA receptors in other brain regions is less well-defined.

Using the receptor binding assay, several studies have been undertaken to search for pharmacologically distinct subclasses of GABA receptor recognition sites. In one study, it was found that while all brain GABA receptors appear to be pharmacologically identical, there does appear to be significant differences with regard to receptor affinity in different brain regions, with GABA receptors in the dentate nucleus having a significantly greater affinity for the ligand than receptors in the cerebellum and cortex (Enna *et al.*, 1978). These differences in receptor affinity may be related to the regional distribution of the 'endogenous modulator(s)'. Further evidence that there may be differences in GABA receptors has been provided by lesioning studies which have shown that the number of high-affinity (20 nM) GABA receptor binding sites can be altered by certain lesions that leave the number of low-affinity (100 nM) binding sites unchanged, suggesting that the membrane, or perhaps cellular, localization of the two sites differ (Guidotti *et al.*, 1979).

2.3.4 Pharmacological characteristics of GABA receptors

A number of electrophysiological and biochemical investigations have been undertaken to define the preferred conformation of GABA receptor agonists and antagonists (Johnston, 1976b; Enna *et al.*, 1977b; Hitzemann and Loh, 1978; Honore *et al.*, 1978; Krogsgaard-Larsen *et al.*, 1978b; Krogsgaard-Larsen and Johnston, 1978; Nicholson *et al.*, 1979). By studying a series of compounds structurally related to muscimol (3-hydroxy-5-aminomethylisoxazole), a potent GABA receptor agonist (Johnston, 1976b), it has been found that the 'active' conformation of GABA for its receptor is partially folded and almost planar. The GABA receptor is stereospecific in that the optical antipodes of 5-(1-aminoethyl)3-isoxazolol have different affinities for the GABA receptor, as do ($\pm$) *cis*- and *trans*-3-aminocyclopentane-1-carboxylic acid (Enna and Snyder, 1977b; Krogsgaard-Larsen *et al.*, 1978a). Based on these observations, new GABA receptor agonists have been synthesized, such as 4,5,6,7-tetrahydroisoxazolo (5,4-*c*) pyridine-3-ol (THIP) a semi-rigid bicyclic isoxazole which appears to be centrally active after systemic administration. While systemically administered muscimol also causes behavioral effects in laboratory animals and man, recent work has indicated that the behavioral and biochemical effects observed after administration of this agent may not be solely due to the presence of muscimol in brain acting at GABA receptors, but rather may be related to the combined action of muscimol and some metabolite or to a metabolite alone (Maggi and Enna, 1979).

Other compounds capable of activating bicuculline-sensitive GABA receptors include 3-aminopropanesulfonic acid, β-guanidinoproprionic acid, imidazole-4-acetic acid, imidazole-4-proprionic acid, *trans*-4-aminocrotonic acid and 4-aminotetrolic acid (Johnston, 1976b). Because of poor lipid solubility, none of these agents is centrally active following systemic administration. Compounds structurally related to GABA but which appear not to be direct-acting receptor agonists include γ-hydroxybutyrate, γ-butyrolactone, 2-pyrrolidone, 2-pyrrolidone acetamide and 1-hydroxy-3-aminopyrrolidone (Enna and Maggi, 1979).

The conformation of the GABA receptor recognition site is also quite selective with regard to antagonists. For example, in the group of phthalideisoquinolines, the (+)-isomer of bicuculline (1S, 9R configuration) is markedly more potent as a receptor antagonist than is the (−)-isomer (1R, 9S configuration) and the (1S, 9S) isomer of hydrastine, is more potent than the (1R, 9R) isomer (Enna *et al.*, 1977b).

In contrast, agents such as picrotoxinin, tetramethylenedisulphotetramine and a series of bicyclophosphates, while potent GABA receptor antagonists electrophysiologically, fail to interact with GABA receptor binding, but are potent in inhibiting picrotoxinin attachment to its membrane binding site (Olsen *et al.*, 1978). Other compounds which appear to act at the ionophore include some convulsant barbiturates, tutin and *p*-chlorophenyl-silatrane (Olsen *et al.*, 1978). These results demonstrate the structural specificity of the GABA receptor site and the pharmacological distinction between the recognition site and the ionophore. No GABA receptor agonists have yet been found which directly activate the ionophore, although there have been suggestions that some barbiturates may act in this way (Olsen *et al.*, 1978).

2.3.5 Benzodiazepines: relationship to GABA and glycine receptors

As outlined above, there is ample electrophysiological evidence to suggest that the benzodiazepines facilitate transmission at inhibitory synapses. Based on biochemical studies, it was hypothesized that benzodiazepines directly activated glycine receptors in the spinal cord (Young *et al.*, 1974). However, this theory has yet to find electrophysiological support (Curtis *et al.*, 1976a). Most of the current electrophysiological data indicate that GABAergic synapses are most sensitive to the benzodiazepines since these drugs are known to enhance presynaptic inhibition in the spinal cord and dorsal column nuclei, and postsynaptic inhibition in dorsal column nuclei, hippocampus, hypothalamus, cerebral cortex and cerebellar cortex (Haefely, 1978). All of these inhibitory actions are thought to be mediated by intrinsic GABAergic neurons. Furthermore, benzodiazepines have been shown to potentiate a GABA inhibitory response in the dorsal raphe (Gallager, 1978), in spinal cord cell cultures (Choi *et al.*, 1977) and to facilitate a behavioral response thought to be mediated by GABA (Waddington, 1978). Other evidence suggesting a GABA hypothesis for the action of the benzodiazepines includes the findings that benzodiazepines are potent in inhibiting convulsions associated with a decrease in GABA receptor activity (Mao *et al.*, 1975; Curtis *et al.*, 1976b), that the benzodiazepines mimic GABAergic drugs with regard to changes in cerebellar cyclic GMP (Biggio *et al.*, 1977a, b) and by the fact that picrotoxin can specifically block some of the behavioral effects of the benzodiazepines (Stein *et al.*, 1975).

This facilitation of GABAergic responses is apparently not due to a direct interaction of benzodiazepines with the GABA receptor recognition site or ionophore since depletion of presynaptic GABA stores prevents the enhancement from occurring (Polc *et al.*, 1974), suggesting an indirect mechanism for the facilitation of transmission. While it has been suggested that benzodiazepines may enhance GABA release or inhibit GABA uptake (Olsen *et al.*, 1977; Mitchell and Martin, 1978), the concentrations necessary to cause these effects are higher than would be predicted on the basis of the potency of these agents. Rather, more recent work has suggested that benzodiazepines facilitate GABAergic transmission by an action at the GABA receptor site.

Thus, biochemical studies of the GABA receptor have revealed that, in brain tissue, there is a Triton-sensitive substance which, when present, significantly lowers the affinity of the receptor recognition site for GABA (Enna and Snyder, 1977b). Subsequent studies have indicated that this substance can modify the affinity of the GABA receptor recognition site in a noncompetitive fashion, possibly by inducing an allosteric change in the conformation of the receptor (Guidotti *et al.*, 1978a). Other experiments have indicated that, like Triton, the benzodiazepines are capable of removing this endogenous substance, which suggests that these drugs may facilitate GABAergic transmission by indirectly enhancing the affinity of the recognition site for GABA (Guidotti *et al.*, 1978a). This substance, termed 'GABA-modulin', appears to be a protein capable of inhibiting both benzodiazepine and GABA receptor binding. Further evidence that there may be some relationship between 'GABA-modulin' and the benzodiazepine receptor was provided by the finding that the phylogenetic development of the Triton-sensitive substance in mammalian central nervous system is quite similar to the phylogenetic development of benzodiazepine receptor sites (Nielsen *et al.*, 1978; Mann and Enna, 1979). Furthermore, following chronic administration of benzodiazepines to rats, there is an alternation in GABA receptor binding in the corpus striatum (Mohler *et al.*, 1978).

Other evidence of an interaction between benzodiazepine and GABA receptors has been obtained by studying the high-affinity binding site for benzodiazepines in brain membranes (Mohler and Okada, 1977b; Squires and Braestrup, 1977). By incubating brain membranes with either muscimol or GABA and a labeled benzodiazepine, it was found that the presence of the GABA receptor agonist increases the affinity of the benzodiazepine receptor for the labeled ligand (Martin and Candy, 1978; Tallman *et al.*, 1978; Karobath and Sperk, 1979; Maurer, 1979). In general, the order of potency of the GABA agonists for enhancing benzodiazepine receptor binding parallels their order of potency as GABA receptor agonists. This activation is stereospecific and it can be blocked by bicuculline (Karobath and Sperk, 1979). However, not all GABA receptor agonists are as potent in activating benzodiazepine binding as would be predicted on the basis of their ability to interact with the GABA receptor. Thus, THIP is active in displacing ^{3}H-GABA from its binding site to brain membranes and is electrophysiologically potent as a GABA agonist (Krogsgaard-Larsen *et al.*, 1977). However, THIP is very weak in activating benzodiazepine binding, and, in fact, will inhibit the muscimol or GABA-induced activation of this binding site which has led to the suggestion that this compound may be a

partial receptor agonist (Braestrup *et al.*, 1980). Other relatively potent
GABA receptor agonists which were weaker than anticipated in activating
benzodiazepine binding include imidazoleacetic acid, piperidine-4-sulfonic
acid and isoguvacine (Braestrup *et al.*, 1980); Maurer, 1979). Thus, the
pharmacological specificity of the GABA receptor which mediates the
activation of benzodiazepine binding sites differs significantly from the
specificity of the sodium-independent GABA receptor site. These findings
suggest that there may indeed be more than one pharmacological type of
GABA receptor in the central nervous system.

As a result of these biochemical studies, models are now being proposed
of the GABA receptor which take into consideration the GABA recognition
site, ionophore, benzodiazepine recognition site and 'GABA-modulin'
(Costa and Guidotti, 1979). However, as pointed out by these authors, these
models, while based on some firm scientific evidence, still require much
more rigorous experimentation before they can be considered definitive.
Thus, though present in neurons, 'GABA-modulin' has not yet been shown
to be localized to GABA synapses under *in vivo* conditions. Similarly, it has
yet to be domonstrated that the activation of benzodiazepine binding by
certain GABA agonists has any functional significance *in vivo*. While these
will be difficult questions to answer, the weight of evidence clearly favors a
GABA receptor hypothesis for the action of benzodiazepines.

2.4   GABA RECEPTOR FUNCTION

2.4.1 Behavioral responses

Inhibition of GABA receptor activity by either receptor blockers, such as
bicuculline or picrotoxin, or by inhibition of GABA synthesis, results in
seizure activity (Horton and Meldrum, 1973; Curtis *et al.*, 1970). On the
other hand, behavioral responses resulting from GABA receptor activation
are less well-defined because of the lack of potent and specific agents which
will activate this receptor system after systemic administration. Nevertheless,
numerous investigations have been conducted in an attempt to classify
GABA receptor-mediated behavior by studying the behavioral response to
GABA, GABA analogues or inhibitors of GABA degradation
(Krogsgaard-Larsen *et al.*, 1979). For example, reports have indicated that
GABA agonists possess anticonvulsant and sedative properties (Meldrum,
1975; Anlezark *et al.*, 1977).

In addition, activation of GABA receptors decreases aggressive behavior
(spontaneous muricide activity) in rat (Delini-Stula and Vassout, 1978), and
it has been reported that GABA agonists antagonize the analgesic action of
morphine and enhance the development of tolerance and physical

dependence to opiates (Ho *et al.*, 1976). Hypothalamic GABA receptors appear to regulate feeding behavior and satiety (Kuryama and Kimura, 1976; Grandison and Guidotti, 1977; Kelly *et al.*, 1977).

Many behavioral studies have been directed towards understanding the functional relationship between GABA receptors and the nigrostriatal dopamine pathway. Thus, physiological, biochemical and pharmacological data suggests that there are descending GABAergic pathways from the neostriatum and globus pallidus to the substantia nigra (Kim *et al.*, 1971; Hattori *et al.*, 1973). An increase in pallidal GABA content results in a reserpine-like akinetic syndrome, an effect which is antagonized by picrotoxin, suggesting that the pallidal GABA fibers exert an inhibitory influence on the nigrostriatal dopamine input (Pycock *et al.*, 1976). However, numerous investigations have suggested that activation of nigral GABA receptors by direct injection of muscimol induces contralateral turning behavior in the rat, which suggests that the GABAergic system tends to disinhibit dopamine neuron firing in the nigra (Oberlander *et al.*, 1977; Scheel-Kruger *et al.*, 1977; Waddington and Cross, 1978). In contrast, it has been reported that intranigral injection of picrotoxin also causes contraversive turning (Tarsy *et al.*, 1975). These conflicting results may be explained by more recent studies which suggest that the turning behavior elicited by the nigral injection of a GABA receptor agonist is dependent upon whether the drug is administered in the rostral or caudal regions of this brain area (James and Starr, 1978). Thus, injections of GABA agonists into the rostral nigra leads to ipsilateral turning, suggesting that GABA is inhibitory on the dopamine output, but injections into the caudal portion of the nigra causes contralateral turning. Importantly, the contralateral turning behavior is not blocked by procedures which inhibit nigrostriatal dopamine cell activity, suggesting that the GABA-induced contralateral movement is probably not mediated through the dopamine system. Accordingly, it would appear that, in the nigra, GABA receptors modulate both dopaminergic and nondopaminergic projections to the corpus striatum.

Systemic administration of muscimol, or agents which inhibit GABA degradation, potentiates neuroleptic-induced catalepsy (Worms and Loyd, 1978). However, intranigral injection of muscimol, or a GABA transaminase inhibitor, antagonizes, whereas injections of muscimol into the globus pallidus potentiates, the neuroleptic-induced catalepsy (Matsui and Kamioka, 1978).

Clearly, activation of GABA receptors leads to a number of behavioral changes. However, the type and intensity of the change depends to a great extent on the method of drug administration and specificity of the drug agent. Until more specific GABA receptor agonists are available, it will be difficult to precisely determine the behavioral consequences of GABA receptor activation.

2.4.2 Biochemical responses

No direct proof has yet been supplied to indicate that GABA receptors are linked to specific enzymes on postsynaptic membranes. However, it seems reasonable to assume that there is some coupling to an enzyme which helps maintain the membrane pump for the transport of Cl^- (Roberts, 1974, Ticku and Olsen, 1977). Possible candidates for this role are the cyclic nucleotides, but *in vitro* experiments have shown that GABA is incapable of activating cyclic nucleotide production at reasonable concentrations (Ferrendelli *et al.*, 1975). However, *in vivo* studies with GABA receptor agonists and antagonists have indicated that the cyclic GMP content of the cerebellar cortex may be under GABAergic control since, when GABA receptor function is inhibited by picrotoxin, the cyclic GMP content in this brain region increases (Biggio *et al.*, 1977b; Mailman *et al.*, 1978). Similarly, the pituitary cyclic AMP content also seems to be modulated by GABAergic receptors in that receptor blockers like bicuculline, or inhibitors of GABA synthesis, cause a significant increase in pituitary levels of this second messenger (Guidotti *et al.*, 1978b).

Interestingly, the benzodiazepines affected cyclic nucleotide production in a manner similar to GABA agonists (Guidotti *et al.*, 1978b). Thus, while these studies do not provide sufficient evidence to conclude that the GABA receptor is directly linked to a cyclic nucleotide generating system, they do indicate that, in some brain areas, the GABA receptor can, at least indirectly, modify the production of these important biochemical constituents.

Since GABA receptors are found in virtually all areas of the brain (Enna, 1979b), it is not surprising to find that modification of GABA receptor activity alters the turnover and release of various other neurotransmitter agents. Thus, activation of GABA receptors has been shown to both inhibit and enhance dopamine release and turnover, depending on the brain area studied and the method of receptor activation (Biswas and Carlsson, 1977; Cheramy *et al.*, 1977, 1978b; Perez de la Mora and Fuxe, 1977; Racagni *et al.*, 1977; Enna *et al.*, 1979; Walters *et al.*, 1979). In addition, GABA receptor activity can modify the concentration of acetylcholine in the corpus striatum (Ladinsky *et al.*, 1976; Javoy *et al.*, 1977; Sethy, 1978) and, *in vitro*, GABA receptor activation has been shown to enhance the release of dopamine from rat brain slices (Giorguieff *et al.*, 1978; Starr, 1978). Undoubtedly GABA receptors modulate the release of other neutrotransmitters, and neuromodulators, either directly or indirectly. A more complete understanding of these interactions will be important in predicting the therapeutic, and side-effect, potential of GABA agonist drugs (Enna *et al.*, 1979).

2.4.3 Hormone regulation

A number of recent studies have indicated that GABA receptors may modulate hormone release. Schally *et al.* (1977) were the first to demonstrate that GABA is capable of inhibiting prolactin release from the anterior pituitary both *in vivo* and *in vitro*. Subsequent studies by a number of workers have found there may be a GABA receptor-mediated enhancement as well as inhibition of prolactin release (Lamberts and Macleod, 1978; Tamminga *et al.*, 1978; Vijayan and McCann, 1978a, 1979; Grandison and Guidotti, 1979; Muller *et al.*, 1979). Whether GABA acts to stimulate or inhibit prolactin secretion in general appears to depend upon whether a GABA receptor agonist is administered centrally or peripherally, although there is by no means a clear-cut distinction based on route of administration (Muller *et al.*, 1979). As a result of these studies it is felt that hypothalamic GABA regulates prolactin release and that there may also be GABA receptors on the anterior pituitary, outside the blood–brain barrier, which can respond to circulating levels of GABA agonists (Grandison and Guidotti, 1979). The enhanced prolactin release resulting from haloperiodol or morphine administration appears to be especially sensitive to inhibition by GABA receptor agonists. In man, it has been reported that systemic administration of muscimol causes a significant elevation in both prolactin and growth hormone release (Tamminga *et al.*, 1978). This effect on growth hormone is similar to what has been reported for rat (Abe *et al.*, 1977). In another study, intraventricular, but not intravenous, administration of GABA in ovariectomized, or in ovariectomized, estrogen and progesterone-treated rats caused an elevation in plasma growth hormone and gonadotrophin levels and a decrease in plasma thyrotropin (Vijayan and McCann, 1978a, b). These authors suggest that this is a centrally mediated phenomenon since *in vitro* incubation of hemipituitaries has no effect on the release of either growth hormone or thyrotropin. Furthermore, bicuculline adminstration had no consistent effect on plasma gonadotrophin, prolactin or thyrotropin levels in ovariectomized rats which prompted these investigators to question the physiological role of GABA in the control of these hormones (Vijayan and McCann, 1978a). Thus, while these early studies are highly suggestive, much work remains to clearly define the role of GABA receptors in the control of adenohypophyseal hormone secretion.

2.4.4 Cardiovascular responses

It has been known for some time that GABA can reduce blood pressure and heart rate in a number of species (Elliott and Hobbinger, 1954; Takahashi *et al.*, 1955). While some investigators claimed that these responses are centrally mediated (Guertzenstein, 1973), others feel that they are primarily due to a peripheral mechanism (Elliott and Hobbinger, 1959). In a more recent series of experiments, Antonaccio and colleagues (Antonaccio and Taylor, 1977; Antonaccio *et al.*, 1978a, b) found that intracerebro-ventricular injection of GABA or muscimol causes a profound reduction in blood pressure, heart rate and renal sympathetic nervous discharge in cat. That this effect was mediated by an activation of central GABA receptors was indicated by the finding that it was reversed by bicuculline and picrotoxin, but not by strychnine (Antonaccio *et al.*, 1978a). Further-more, it was also demonstrated that muscimol, administered in this way, causes a significant inhibition of the pressor response elicited by electrical diencephalic stimulation, which was most likely mediated by a reduction in centrally emanating sympathetic discharge to vasoconstrictor nerves (Antonaccio *et al.*, 1978b). These results indicate that brain GABA receptor activation can reduce sympathetic nerve activity, which in turn causes a reduction in blood pressure and heart rate. However, from this work, it is not possible to determine the precise location of the GABA receptors in brain which mediate this action.

On the other hand, GABA receptors have been located on neurons in the nucleus ambiguous of the brainstem, and these appear to regulate vagal outflow (Dimicco *et al.*, 1979). Evidence for this is provided by the report that microinjection of bicuculline, or an inhibitor of GABA synthesis, into this nucleus causes a significant, dose-dependent reduction in heart rate and blood pressure. Interestingly, while muscimol was able to reverse the bicuculline-induced bradycardia and hypotension, it has no effect on either parameter when placed alone into the nucleus ambiguous suggesting that the GABA receptors in this area are normally fully activated.

Thus, GABA receptors may play an important role in the central regulation of the cardiovascular system. Accordingly, pharmacological manipulation of these receptors may represent a new approach for the therapy of some cardiovascular disorders.

2.5 SUMMARY

GABA and glycine are potent inhibitory transmitters in the central nervous system. Activation of the neuronal receptors for either of these amino acids produces a postsynaptic IPSP which is mediated by a transient increase in Cl^- conductance. Despite this commonality, there are numerous differences between the GABA and glycine receptor systems. Thus GABA receptors mediate postsynaptic inhibition throughout the central nervous system, whereas glycine receptors are found primarily in the spinal cord and brain stem. Furthermore, GABA, but not glycine, receptors may also be localized presynaptically in the spinal cord and GABA, but not glycine, receptors can be desensitized. Finally, the receptors for the two neurotransmitters are pharmacologically distinct.

With regard to GABA, both biochemical and electrophysiological studies suggest that there may be a number of GABA receptor sites. There may be two types of receptor recognition site, each with a different affinity for GABA, which, while pharmacologically indistinct, may regulate different systems. In addition, the recognition site may have two different conformations, an agonist and an antagonist, as has been suggested for other transmitter receptors. Furthermore, the ionophore associated with GABA or glycine receptors appears to be distinct, but intimately related to, the recognition site. Finally, the potential existence of an 'endogenous modulator(s)' of the GABA receptor, while contributing to the complexity of this system, may be a target for drugs, such as the benzodiazepines, which can regulate GABA receptor activity. Thus, the GABA and glycine receptors should probably not be thought of as singular entities, but rather, as a family of sites, some of which function in concert, some of which are independent, with the final effect of receptor activation, or inhibition, being dependent upon which site, or combination of sites, is involved.

REFERENCES

Abe, H., Kato, Y., Chihara, K., Ohgo, S., Owasaki, S. and Imura, H. (1977), *Endocrinol. Jap.*, **24**, 229–233.

Adams, P.R. and Brown, D.A. (1973), *Brit. J. Pharmac.*, **47**, 639–640.

Adams, P.R. and Brown, D.A. (1975), *J. Physiol., (Lond.)*, **250**, 85–120.

Anlezark, G., Collins, J. and Meldrum, B. (1977), *Neurosci. Lett.*, **7**, 337–340.

Antonaccio, M., Kerwin, L. and Taylor, D. (1978a), *Neuropharmac.*, **17**, 783–791.

Antonaccio, M., Kerwin, L. and Taylor, D. (1978b), *Neuropharmac.*, **17**, 597–603.

Antonaccio, M. and Taylor, D. (1977), *Europ. J. Pharmac.*, **46**, 283–287.

Aprison, M.H. (1970), *Pharmacologist*, **12**, 222.

Aprison, M.H. and Werman, R. (1965), *Life Sci.*, **4**, 2075–2083.

Araki, T., Ito, M. and Oscarsson, O. (1961), *J. Physiol.*, **159**, 410–435.

Barker, J.L. and Nicoll, R.A. (1972), *Science*, **176**, 1043–1045.

Barker, J.L., Nicoll, R.A. and Padjen, A. (1975), *J. Physiol., (Lond.)*, **245**, 521–536.

Barron, D.H. and Matthews, B.H.C. (1938), *J. Physiol., (Lond.)*, **92**, 276–321.

Beaumont, K., Chilton, W.S., Yamamura, H.I. and Enna, S.J. (1978), *Brain Res.*, **148**, 153–162.

Biggio, G., Brodie, B.B., Costa, E. and Guidotti, A. (1977a), *Proc. natn. Acad. Sci. USA*, **174**, 3592–3596.

Biggio, G., Costa, E. and Guidotti, A. (1977b), *J. Pharmac. exp. Therap.*, **200**, 207–215.

Biswas, B. and Carlsson, A. (1977), *N-S Arch. Pharmac.*, **299**, 41–46.

Bowery, N.G. and Brown, D.A. (1974), *Brit. J. Pharmac.*, **50**, 205–218.

Braestrup, C., Nielsen, M., and Krogsgaard-Larsen, P. (1980), *Receptors for Neurotransmitters and Peptide Hormones*. (Pepeu, G., Kuhar, M.J., and Enna, S.J., eds), Raven Press, New York. pp. 301–312.

Bridgers, W.R. (1965), *J. biol. Chem.*, **240**, 4591–4597.

Brock, L.G., Coombs, J.S. and Eccles, J.C. (1952), *J. Physiol.*, **117**, 8P.

Brooks, N. and Werman, R. (1973), *Mol. Pharmac.*, **9**, 571–579.

Chan-Palay, V. (1978), *Proc. natn. Acad. Sci. USA*, **75**, 1024–1028.

Cheramy, A., Nieoullon, A. and Glowinski, J. (1977), *N-S Arch. Pharmac.*, **297**, 31–37.

Cheramy, A., Nieoullon, A. and Glowinski, J. (1978a), *Europ. J. Pharmac.*, **47**, 141–147.

Cheramy, A., Nieoullon, A. and Glowinski, J. (1978b), *Europ. J. Pharmac.* **48**, 281–295.

Choi, D.W., Farb, D.H. and Fischbach, G.D. (1977), *Nature*, **269**, 342–344.

Christensen, H.N. (1973), *Proc. Am. Soc. exp. Biol.*, **32**, 19–28.

Coombs, J.S., Eccles, J.C. and Fatt, P. (1955), *J. Physiol.*, **130**, 326–373.

Costa, E. and Guidotti, A. (1974), *Ann. Rev. Pharmac. Toxicol.*, **19**, 531–545.

Costa, E., Guidotti, A. and Mao, C.C. (1975), *Adv. Biochem. Psychopharmac.* **14**, 113–130.

Coyle, J.T. and Enna, S.J. (1976), *Brain Res.*, **111**, 119–133.

Crossman, A.R., Walker, R.J. and Woodruff, G.N. (1973), *Brit. J. Pharmac.*, **49**, 696–698.

Curtis, D.R. and Duggan, A.W. (1969), *Agents and Actions*, **1**, 14–19.

Curtis, D.R. and Johnston, G.A.R. (1974a), *Ergeb Physiol.*, **69**, 98–165.

Curtis, D.R. and Johnston, G.A.R. (1975b), *Neuropoisons*. (Simpson, L.L. and Curtis, D.R, eds) Plenum Press, New York. pp. 207–248.

Curtis, D.R., Duggan, A.W., Felix, D. and Johnston, G.A.R. (1970), *Nature (Lond.)* **226**, 1222–1224.

Curtis, D.R., Game, C.J. and Lodge, D. (1976a), *Brit. J. Pharmac.*, **56**, 307–311.

Curtis, D.R., Hosli, L., and Johnston, G.A.R. (1968a), *Exp. Brain Res.*, **6**, 1–18.

Curtis, D.R., Hosli, L., Johnston, G.A.R. and Johnston, I.H. (1967), *Brain Res.*, **5**, 112–114.

Curtis, D.R., Hosli, L., Johnston, G.A.R. and Johnston, I.H. (1968b), *Exp. Brain Res.*, **5**, 235–258.

Curtis, D.R., Lodge, D., Johnston, G.A.R. and Brand, S.J. (1976b), *Brain Res.*, **118**, 344–347.

Curtis, D.R., Phillis, J.W. and Watkins, J.C. (1959), *J. Physiol.*, **146**, 185–203.

Curtis, D.R., Phillis, J.W. and Watkins, J.C. (1960), *J. Physiol.*, **150**, 656–682.

Curtis, D.R. and Tebēcis, A.K. (1972), *Exp. Brain Res.*, **16**, 210–218.

Davidoff, R.A. (1977), *Science*, **75**, 331–333.

Davidoff, R.A., Graham, L.T., Shank, R.P. Werman, R. and Aprison, M.H. (1967a), *J. Neurochem.*, **14**, 1025–1031.

Davidoff, R.A., Schank, R.P., Graham, L.T., Aprison, M.H. and Werman, R. (1967b), *Nature*, **214**, 680–681.

Davidson, N. (1976), *Neurotransmitter Amino Acids.* Academic Press, New York.

DeFeudis, F.V. (1973), *Exp. Neurol.*, **41**, 54–62.

DeFeudis, F.V. (1975), *Ann. Rev. Pharmac.*, **15**, 105–130.

de Groat, W.C. (1972), *Brain Res.*, **18**, 429–432.

Delini-Stula, A. and Vassout, A. (1978), *Neuropharmac.*, **17**, 1063–1065.

Deschenes, M., Feltz, P. and Lamoni, Y. (1976), *Brain Res.*, **118**, 486–493.

Dimicco, J., Gale, K., Hamilton, B. and Gillis, R.A. (1979), *Science,* **204,** 1106–1109.

Douglas, G.W. and Martensen, R.A. (1956), *J. biol. Chem.,* **222,** 581–585.

Dray, A. and Gonye, T.J. (1975), *J. Physiol.* (Lond.), **246,** 22P–23P.

Dray, A., Gonye, T.J. and Oakely, N.R. (1976), *J. Physiol. (Lond.),* **259,** 825–849.

Dreifuss, J.J., Kelly, J.S. and Krnjevic, K. (1969), *Exp. Brain Res.,* **9,** 137–154.

Eccles, J.C. (1964), *The Physiology of Synapses.* Springer-Verlag, Berlin.

Eccles, J.C., Eccles, R.M. and Ito, M. (1964a), *Proc. R. Soc. Brit.,* **160,** 181–196.

Eccles, J.C., Eccles, R.M. and Ito, M. (1964b), *Proc. R. Soc. Brit.,* **160,** 197–210.

Eccles, J.C., Schmidt, R.F. and Willis, W.D. (1962), *J. Physiol.,* **1961,** 282–297.

Eccles, J.C., Schmidt, R.F. and Willis, W.D. (1963), *J. Physiol.,* **168,** 500–530.

Elliott, K. and Hobbinger, F. (1959), *J. Physiol.,* **146,** 70–84.

Enna, S.J. (1979a), *Ann. Rep. Med. Chem.,* **14,** 41–50.

Enna, S.J. (1979b), *GABA- Biochemistry and CNS Function.* (Mandel, P., DeFeudis, F.V. and Mark, J., eds), Plenum Press, pp. 323–337.

Enna, S.J. and Maggi, A. (1979), *Life Sci.,* **24,** 1727–1738.

Enna, S.J. and Snyder, S.H. (1975), *Brain Res.,* **100,** 81–97.

Enna, S.J. and Snyder, S.H. (1976), *Brain Res.,* **115,** 174–179.

Enna, S.J. and Snyder, S.H. (1977a), *J. Neurochem.,* **28,** 857–860.

Enna, S.J. and Snyder, S.H. (1977b), *Mol. Pharmac.,* **13,** 442–453.

Enna, S.J., Bennett, J.P., Bylund, D.B., Creese, I., Burt, D.R., Charness, M.E., Yamamura, H.I., Simantov, R. and Snyder, S.H. (1977a), *J. Neurochem.,* **28,** 233–236.

Enna, S.J., Collins, J.F. and Snyder, S.H. (1977b), *Brain Res.,* **124,** 185–190.

Enna, S.J., Ferkany, J.W. and Krogsgaard-Larsen, P. (1978), *GABA-Neurotransmitters.* (Kofod, H., Krogsgaard-Larsen, P. and Scheel-Kruger, J., eds), Munksgaard, Copenhagen. pp. 191–200.

Enna, S.J., Ferkany, J.W. and Strong, R. (1979), *Receptors for Neurotransmitter and Peptide Hormones.* (Pepeu, G., Kuhar, M.J. and Enna, S.J., eds), Raven Press, New York, pp. 253–263.

Enna, S.J., Kuhar, M.J. and Snyder, S.H. (1975), *Brain Res.,* **93,** 168–174.

Enna, S.J., Yamamura, H.I. and Snyder, S.H. (1976), *Brain Res.,* **101,** 177–183.

Fahn, S. (1976), *GABA in Nervous System Function.* (Roberts, E., Chase, T.N. and Tower, D.B., eds), Raven Press, New York. pp. 169–186.

Ferrendelli, J.A., Ratcheson, R.A. and Kinscherf, D.A. (1979), *Proc. Am. Soc. Neurochem.,* **6,** 78.

Fonnum, F. (1978), *Amino Acids as Chemical Transmitters.* Plenum Press, New York.

Frank, K. (1959), *IRE, Inst. Radio Engrs. Trans. Med. Electron,* **ME-6,** 85–88.

Frank, K. and Fuortes, M.G.F. (1957), *Fed. Proc.,* **16,** 39–40.

Gallager, D.W. (1978), *Europ. J. Pharmacol.* **49,** 133–143.

Giorguieff, M.F., Kemel, M.L. Glowinski, J. and Besson, M.J. (1978), *Brain Res.,* **139,** 115–130.

Globus, A., Lux, H.D. and Schubert, P. (1968), *Brain Res.,* **11,** 440–445.

Gottesfeld, Z. and Elliott, K.A.C. (1971), *J. Neurochem.,* **18,** 683–690.

Graham, L.T., Shank, R.P., Werman, R. and Aprison, M.H. (1967), *J. Neurochem.,* **14,** 465–472.

Grandison, L. and Guidotti, A. (1977), *Neuropharmac.,* **16**, 533–536.

Grandison, L. and Guidotti, A. (1979), *Endocrinology,* **105**, 754–759.

Greenlee, D.V., Van Ness, P.C. and Olsen, R.W. (1978a), *J. Neurochem.,* **31**, 933–938.

Greenlee, D.V., Van Ness, P.C. and Olsen, R.W. (1978b), *Life Sci.,* **22**, 1653–1662.

Guerzenstein, P.G. (1973), *J. Physiol. Lond.,* **229**, 395–408.

Guidotti, A., Gale, K., Suria, A. and Toffano, G. (1979), *Brain Res.,* **172**, 566–571.

Guidotti, A., Toffano, G. and Costa, E. (1978a), *Nature,* **257**, 553–555.

Guidotti, A., Toffano, G., Grandison, L. and Costa, E. (1978b), *Amino Acids as Chemical Transmitters.* (Fonnum F., ed), Plenum Press, New York. pp. 517–530.

Haas, L. and Hosli, L. (1973), *Brain Res.,* **52**, 399–402.

Haefely, W.E. (1978), *Brit. J. Psychiat.,* **133**, 231–238.

Haefely, W.E., Kulcsai, A., Mohler, H., Piere, L., Polc, P. and Schaffner, R. (1975), *Adv. Biochem. Psychopharmac.,* **14**, 131–139.

Hammerstad, J.P., Murry, J.E. and Cutler, R.W.P. (1971), *Brain Res.,* **35**, 357–367.

Hattori, T., McGeer, P.L., Fibiger, H.C. and McGeer, E.G. (1973), *Brain Res.,* **54**, 103–114.

Henn, F.A. and Hamberger, A. (1971), *Proc. natn. Acad. Sci., USA,* **68**, 2686–2690.

Hitzemann, R.J. and Loh, H.H. (1978), *Brain Res.,* **144**, 63–73.

Ho, I.K., Loh, H.H. and Way, E.L. (1976), *Life Sci.,* **18**, 1111–1124.

Honore, T., Hjeds, H., Krogsgaard-Larsen, P. and Christiansen, R. (1978), *Europ. J. Med. Chem.,* **13**, 429–434.

Hopkins, J.M. and Neal, M.J. (1970), *Brit. J. Pharmac.,* **4**, 136P–138P.

Horton, R.W. and Meldrum, B.S. (1973), *Brit. J. Pharmac.,* **49**, 52–63.

Hosli, L. and Tebēcis, A.K. (1970), *Exp. Brain Res.,* **11**, 111–127.

Iversen, L.L. and Bloom, F.E. (1972), *Brain Res.,* **41**, 131–143.

Iversen, L.L. and Neal, M.J. (1968), *J. Neurochem.,* **15**, 1141–1149.

James, T.A. and Starr, M.S. (1978), *Nature,* **275**, 229–230.

Javoy, F., Euvrard, C., Herbet, A. and Glowinski, J. (1977), *Brain Res.,* **126**, 382–386.

Johnston, G.A.R. (1976a), *Chemical Transmission in the Central Nervous System.* (S.H. Hockman and D. Buger, eds), University Park Press, Baltimore. pp. 31–81.

Johnston, G.A.R. (1976b), *GABA in Nervous System Function.* (Roberts, E., Chase, T.N. and Tower, D.B., eds), Raven Press, New York. pp. 395–411.

Johnston, G.A.R. and Iversen, L.L. (1971), *J. Neurochem.,* **18**, 1951–1961.

Johnston, G.A.R. and Kennedy, S.M.E. (1978), *Amino Acids as Chemical Transmitters.* (Fonnum, F., ed), Plenum Press, New York. pp. 507–516.

Johnston, G.A.R., Vitali, M.V. and Alexander, H.M. (1970), *Brain Res.,* **20**, 361–367.

Karobath, M. and Sperk, G. (1979), *Proc. natn. Acad. Sci., USA,* **76**, 1004–1006.

Katz, B. and Thesleff, S. (1957), *J. Physiol. (Lond.),* **138**, 63–80.

Kelly, J., Alheid, G.F., Newberg, A. and Grossman, S.P. (1977), *Pharmac. Biochem. Behav.,* **7**, 537–541.

Kim, J.S., Bak, I.J., Hassler, R. and Okada, Y. (1971), *Exp. Brain Res.,* **14**, 95–104.

Krnjevic, R. and Morris, M.E. (1974), *Can. J. Physiol. Pharmac.,* **52**, 852–871.

Krnjevic, K. and Morris, M.E. (1975), *Can. J. Physiol. Pharmac.*, **53**, 912–922.
Krnjevic, K. and Phillis, J.W. (1963), *J. Physiol.*, **165**, 274–304.
Krnjevic, K. and Schwartz, S. (1966), *Nature (Lond.)*, **211**, 1372–1374.
Krnjevic, K. and Schwartz, S. (1967), *Exp. Brain Res.*, **3**, 306–319.
Krnjevic, K., Puil, E. and Werman, R. (1977a), *Can. J. Physiol. Pharmac.*, **55**, 658–669.
Krnjevic, K., Puil, E. and Werman, R. (1977b), *Can. J. Physiol. Pharmac.*, **55**, 670–680.
Krogsgaard-Larsen, P. and Johnston, G.A.R. (1978), *J. Neurochem.*, **30**, 1377–1382.
Krogsgaard-Larsen, P., Honore, T. and Thyssen, K. (1978a), *GABA-Neurotransmitters*. (Kofod, H., Krogsgaard-Larsen, P. and Scheel-Kruger, J., eds), Munksgaard, Copenhagen. pp. 201–216.
Krogsgaard-Larsen, P., Johnston, G.A.R., Lodge, D. and Curtis, D.R. (1977), *Nature*, **268**, 53–55.
Krogsgaard-Larsen, P., Nordahl, A. and Thyssen, K. (1978b), *Acta Chem. Scand.*, **32**, 469–477.
Krogsgaard-Larsen, P., Scheel-Kruger, J. and Kofod, H. (1979), *GABA-Neurotransmitters*. Munksgaard, Copenhagen.
Kuhar, M.J., Green, A.I., Snyder, S.H. and Gfeller, E. (1970), *Brain Res.*, **21**, 405–417.
Kuhar, M.J., Shaskan, E.G. and Snyder, S.H. (1971), *J. Neurochem.*, **18**, 333–343.
Kuriyama, K. and Kimura, H. (1976), *GABA in Nervous System Function* (Roberts, E., Chase, T. and Tower, D.B., eds), Raven Press, New York. pp. 203–216.
Kuriyama, K., Roberts, E. and Vos, J. (1968), *Brain Res.*, **9**, 231–252.
Ladinsky, H., Consolo, S., Bianchi, S. and Jori, A. (1976), *Brain Res.*, **108**, 351–361.
Lamberts, S. and MacLeod, R. (1978), *Proc. Soc. exp. Biol. Med.*, **158**, 10–13.
Laris, P.C., Pershadsingh, H.A., and Johnstone, R.M. (1976), *Biochem. Biophys. Acta*, **436**, 475–488.
Leach, M.J. and Wilson, J.A. (1978), *Europ. J. Pharmac.*, **48**, 329–330.
LeFort, D., Henke, H. and Cuenod, M. (1978), *J. Neurochem.*, **30**, 1287–1291.
Lester, B.R. and Peck, E.J. (1979), *Brain Res.*, **161**, 79–97.
Lloyd, D.P.C. (1941), *J. Neurophysiol.*, **4**, 184–190.
Logan, W.J. and Snyder, S.H. (1972), *Brain Res.*, **42**, 413–431.
Lothman, E.W. and Somjen, G.G. (1975), *J. Physiol. (Lond.)*, **252**, 115–136.
MacDonald, R. and Bacher, J.L. (1978), *Nature*, **271**, 563–564.
MacKerer, C.R., Kochman, R.L., Shen, T.F. and Hershenson, F.M. (1977), *J. Pharmac. exp. Therap.*, **201**, 326–331.
Maggi, A. and Enna, S.J. (1979), *Neuropharmac.*, **18**, 361–366.
Mailman, R.B., Mueller, R.A. and Breese, G.R. (1978), *Life Sci.*, **23**, 623–628.
Mann, E. and Enna, S.J. (1979), *Brain Res.*, in press.
Mao, C.C., Guidotti, A. and Costa, E. (1975), *N-S Arch. Pharmac.*, **284**, 369–378.
Martin, I.L. and Candy, J.M. (1978), *Neuropharmac.*, **17**, 993–958.
Mase, K., Takahashi, U. and Ogata, K. (1962), *J. Neurochem.*, **9**, 281–288.
Matsui, Y. and Kamioka, T. (1978), *N-S Arch. Pharmac.*, **305**, 219–225.
Matus, A.I. and Dennison, M.E. (1971), *Brain Res.*, **32**, 195–197.
Maurer, R. (1979), *Neurosci. Lett.*, **12**, 65–68.

McLaughlin, B.J., Wood, J.G., Saito, K., Barber, R., Vaughn, J., Roberts, E. and Wu, J. (1974), *Brain Res.*, **76**, 377–391.

Meldrum, B.S. (1975), *Int. Rev. Neurobiol.*, **17**, 1–36.

Mitchell, P.R. and Martin, I.L. (1978), *Neuropharmac.*, **17**, 317–320.

Mohler, H. and Okada, T. (1977a), *Nature*, **267**, 65–67.

Mohler, H. and Okada, T. (1977b), *Life Sci.*, **20**, 2101–2110.

Mohler, H. and Okada, T. (1978), *Mol. Pharmac.*, **14**, 256–265.

Mohler, H., Okada, T. and Enna, S.J. (1978), *Brain Res.*, **156**, 391–395.

Muller, E.E., Cocchi, D., Lacatelli, V., Krogsgaard-Larsen, P., Bruno, F. and Racagni, G. (1979), *GABA-Neurotransmitters*. (Krogsgaard-Larsen, P., Scheel-Kruger, J. and Kofod, H., eds), Munksgaard, Copenhagen. pp. 518–532.

Muller, W.E. and Snyder, S.H. (1978a), *Brain Res.*, **143**, 487–498.

Muller, W.E. and Snyder, S.H. (1978b), *Brain Res.*, **147**, 107–116.

Neal, M.J. and Pickles, H.G. (1969), *Nature*, **222**, 679–680.

Nicholson, S.H., Suckling, C.J. and Iversen, L.L. (1979), *J. Neurochem.*, **32**, 249–252.

Nielsen, M., Braestrup, C. and Squires, R. (1978), *Brain Res.*, **141**, 342–346.

Nishi, S., Minota, S. and Karozman, A.G. (1974), *Neuropharmac.*, **13**, 215–219.

Obata, K. (1972), *Fed. Proc.*, **31**, 231.

Oberlander, C., Dumont, C. and Boissier, J. (1977), *Eur. J. Pharmac.*, **43**, 389–390.

Olsen, R.W., Lamar, E.E. and Bayless, J.D. (1977), *J. Neurochem.*, **28**, 299–305.

Olsen, R.W., Ticku, M.K., Greenlee, D. and Van Ness, P. (1978), *GABA-Neurotransmitters*. (Kofod, H., Krogsgaard-Larsen, P. and Scheel-Kruger, J., eds), Munksgaard, Copenhagen. pp. 165–178.

Oomura, Y., Sawada, M., Tanikawa, T. and Ooyama, H. (1974), *Nature (Lond.)*, **250**, 258–260.

Osborne, R.H., Bradford, H.F. and Jones, D.G. (1973), *J. Neurochem.*, **21**, 407–419.

Otsuka, M. and Konishi, S. (1976), *GABA in Nervous System Function*, Vol. 5. (Roberts, E., Chase, T.N. and Tower, D.B., eds), Raven Press, New York. pp. 197–202.

Palacios, J.M., Young, W.S. and Kuhar, M.J. (1980), *Proc. natn. Acad. Sci. USA*, **77**, 670–674.

Perez de la Mora, M. and Fuxe, K. (1977), *Brain Res.*, **135**, 107–122.

Phillis, J.W. and York, D.H. (1967), *Nature (Lond.)*, **216**, 922–923.

Phillis, J.W. and York, D.H. (1968a), *Life Sci. (Oxford)*, **7**, 65–69.

Phillis, J.W. and York, D.H. (1968b), *Brain Res.*, **10**, 297–306.

Phillis, J.W., Tebecis, A.K. and York, D.H. (1968), *Brit. J. Pharmac.*, **33**, 426–440.

Polc, P., Mohler, H. and Haefely, W. (1974), *Arch. Pharmac.*, **284**, 319–337.

Pycock, C., Horton, R.W. and Marsden, C.D. (1976), *Brain Res.*, **116**, 353–359.

Racagni, G., Bruno, F., Cattabeni, F., Maggi, A., DiGiulio, A., Parenti, M. and Gropetti, A. (1977), *Brain Res.*, **134**, 353–358.

Ransom, B.R. and Barker, J.L. (1976), *Brain Res.*, **114**, 530–535.

Redburn, D.A., Broome, D., Fekany, J. and Enna, S.J. (1978), *Brain Res.*, **152**, 511–519.

Roberts, E. (1974), *Biochem. Pharmac.*, **23**, 2637–2649.

Roberts, E. and Frankel, S. (1950), *J. biol. Chem.*, **187**, 55–63.

Roberts, E. and Hammerschlag, R. (1976), *Basic Neurochemistry*. (Seigel, G.J., Albers, R.W., Katzman, R. and Agranoff, B.W., eds), Little, Brown, Boston. pp. 218–245.

Roberts, E. and Kuriyama, K. (1968), *Brain Res.*, **8**, 1–35.

Roberts, P.J. and Mitchell, J.F. (1972), *J. Neurochem.*, **19**, 2473–2481.

Rose, R.C. and Schultz, S.G. (1970), *Biochem. biophys. Acta*, **211**, 376–378.

Schally, A.V., Redding, T.W., Arimura, A., Dupont, A. and Linthicum, G. (1977), *Endocrinology*, **100**, 681–691.

Scheel-Kruger, J., Arnt, J. and Magelund, G. (1977), *Neurosci. Lett.*, **4**, 351–356.

Schon, F., Beart, P.M., Chapman, D. and Kelly, J.S. (1975), *Brain Res.*, **85**, 479–490.

Schultz, S.G. and Curran, P.F. (1970), *Physiol. Rec.*, **50**, 637–718.

Sethy, V.H. (1978), *Res. Comm. chem. Path. Pharmac.*, **21**, 359–362.

Simantov, R., Oster-Granite, M.L., Herndon, R. and Snyder, S.H. (1976), *Brain Res.*, **105**, 365–371.

Snodgrass, S.R. (1978), *Nature*, **273**, 392–394.

Squires, R. and Braestrup, C. (1977), *Nature*, **266**, 732–734.

Starr, M.S. (1978), *Europ. J. Pharmac.*, **48**, 325–328.

Stein, L., Wise, C.D. and Belluzzi, J. (1975), *Mechanism of Action of Benzodiazepines*. (Costa, E. and Greengard, P., eds), Raven Press, New York. pp. 29–44.

Tallman, J.F., Thomas, J.W. and Gallager, D.W. (1978), *Nature*, **274**, 383–385.

Takahashi, H., Tiba, M., Ino, M. and Takayasu, T. (1955), *Jap. J. Physiol.*, **5**, 334–339.

Tamminga, C., Neophytides, A., Chase, T. and Frohman, L. (1978), *J. clin. Endocrin. Metab.*, **47**, 1348–1351.

Tarsy, D., Pycock, C., Meldrum, B. and Marsden, C.D. (1975), *Brain Res.*, **89**, 160–165.

ten Bruggencate, G. and Engberg, I. (1968), *Brain Res.*, **11**, 446–450.

Ticku, M.K. and Olsen, R.W. (1977), *Biochem. Biophys. Acta.*, **464**, 519–529.

Ticku, M.K. and Olsen, R.W. (1978), *Life Sci.*, **22**, 1643–1652.

Ticku, M.K., Van Ness, P.C., Haycock, J.W., Levy, W.B. and Olsen, R.W. (1978), *Brain Res.*, 642–647.

Toffano, G., Leon, A., Massotti, M., Guidotti, A. and Costa, E. (1980), *Receptors for Hormones and Neurotransmitters*, G. Pepeu, M.J. Kuhar and S.J. Enna (eds), Raven Press, New York, pp. 133–142.

Toffano, G., Guidotti, A. and Costa, E. (1978), *Proc. natn. Acad. Sci. USA*, **75**, 4024–4028.

Uhr, M.L. and Sneddon, M.K. (1972), *J. Neurochem.*, **19**, 1495–1500.

Varon, S., Weinstein, H., Kakefuda, T. and Roberts, E. (1965), *Biochem. Pharmac.*, **14**, 1213–1224.

Vijayan, E. and McCann, S. (1978a), *Brain Res.*, **155**, 35–43.

Vijayan, E. and McCann, S. (1978b), *Endocrinol.*, **103**, 1888–1893.

Vijayan, E. and McCann, S. (1979), *Brain Res.*, **162**, 69–76.

Waddington, J.L. (1978), *Europ. J. Pharmac.*, **51**, 417–422.

Waddington, J.L. and Cross, A.J. (1978), *Nature*, **276**, 618–620.

Walters, J.R., Lakoski, J.M., Eng., N. and Waszczak, B.L. (1979),

GABA-Neurotransmitters. (Krogsgaard-Larsen, P., Scheel-Kruger, J. and Kofod, H., eds), 134, Munksgaard, Copenhagen. pp. 118–134.

Weight, F.F. (1974), *The Neurosciences. Third Study Program.* (Schmidt, F.O. and Worden, F.G., eds), MIT Press, Boston. pp. 929–941.

Weight, F.F. and Frulkar, S.D. (1976), *Science,* **193**, 1023–1025.

Werman, R. (1975), *Stability and Origin of Biological Information.* (Miller, I.R., ed) Witz, New York. pp. 226–244.

Werman, R. and Aprison, M.H. (1968), *Structure and Function of Inhibitory Neuronal Mechanisms.* (Von Euler, C., Skogland, S. and Soderberg, V., eds), Pergamon Press, Oxford. pp. 473–486.

Werman, R. Davidoff, R.A. and Aprison, M.H. (1967), *Nature (Lond.),* **214**, 681–683.

Werman, R., Davidoff, R.A. and Aprison, M.H., (1968), *J. Neurophysiol.,* **31**, 81–95.

Winkler, M.H., Nicklas, W.J. and Berl, S. (1979), *J. Neurochem.,* **32**, 79–84.

Worms, P. and Lloyd, K.G. (1978), *Life Sci.,* **23**, 475–478.

Wong, D.T. and Horng, J.S. (1977), *Life Sci.,* **20**, 445–452.

Young, A.B. and Snyder, S.H. (1973). *Proc. natn. Acad. Sci. USA,* **70**, 2832–2836.

Young, A.B. and Snyder, S.H. (1974a), *Mol. Pharmac.,* **10**, 790–809.

Young, A.B. and Snyder, S.H. (1974b), *Proc. natn. Acad. Sci. USA,* **71**, 4002–4005.

Young, A.B., Zukin, S.R. and Snyder, S.H. (1974), *Proc. natn. Acad. Sci., USA,* **71**, 2246–2250.

Zukin, S.R., Young, A.B. and Snyder, S.H. (1974), *Proc. natn. Acad. Sci., USA,* **71**, 4802–4807.

3 Substance P Receptors

MICHAEL R. HANLEY and LESLIE L. IVERSEN

Acknowledgement
M.R.H. is a postdoctoral Fellow of the Helen Whitney Foundation.

Neurotransmitter Receptors Part 1
(*Receptors and Recognition*, Series B, Volume 9)
Edited by S.J. Enna and H.I. Yamamura
Published in 1980 by Chapman and Hall, 11 New Fetter Lane,
London EC4P 4EE
© Chapman and Hall

3.1 INTRODUCTION

Substance P (SP) is an undecapeptide with powerful spasmogenic activity on smooth muscle originally identified in extracts of equine intestine by von Euler and Gaddum (1931). The peptide was later isolated from hypothalamus and characterized by Chang and Leeman (1970) and Chang *et al.* (1971), and from intestine by Studer *et al.* (1973). It belongs to a family of related peptides with rapid stimulant actions on vascular and extravascular smooth muscle, known as the *tachykinins* (Erspamer and Anastasi, 1966) (Table 3.1). SP is the only such mammalian peptide, the others being of amphibian origin, except for eledoisin which occurs in octopus salivary gland.

The availability of synthetic SP has allowed the development of sensitive immunohistochemical and immunoassay techniques, and a considerable amount of information is now available on the distribution of this peptide in the nervous system and peripheral tissues. There is substantial evidence that SP may act as a peptide neurotransmitter in the mammalian CNS. It appears to be one of the sensory transmitters released from primary afferent fibres, and is also present within a number of intrinsic neuronal pathways within the brain. The evidence for the hypothesis of a neurotransmitter role for SP has been reviewed in detail elsewhere (Leeman and Mroz, 1974; Otsuka and Konishi, 1976; von Euler and Pernow, 1977; Cuello *et al.*, 1978; Skrabanek and Powell, 1978).

This chapter will focus on the receptor mechanisms which mediate biological responses to SP in neural and non-neural tissues. Although SP

Table 3.1 Structures of tachykinins.

	1	2	3	4	5	6	7	8	9	10	11
Substance P	Arg-	Pro-	Lys-	Pro-	Gln-	Gln-	Phe*-	Phe-	Gly*-	Leu*-	Met*-NH$_2$
Phyllomedusin	pGlu†-	Asn-	Pro-	Asn-	Arg-	Phe*-	Ile-	Gly*-	Leu*-	Met*-NH$_2$	
Eledoisin	pGlu†-	Pro-	Ser-	Lys-	Asp-	Ala-	Phe*-	Ile-	Gly*-	Leu*-	Met*-NH$_2$
Physalaemin	pGlu†-	Ala-	Asp-	Pro-	Asn-	Lys-	Phe*-	Tyr-	Gly*-	Leu*-	Met*-NH$_2$
Uperolein	pGlu†-	Pro-	Asp-	Pro-	Asn-	Ala-	Phe*-	Tyr-	Gly*-	Leu*-	Met*-NH$_2$
Kassinin	Asp-	Val-	Pro-	Lys-	Ser-	Asp-	Gln-	Phe*-	Val-	Gly*-	Leu*-Met*-NH$_2$

* Conserved residues.
† pGlu-pyroglutamic acid.

73

Table 3.2 Relative potencies of substance P fragments on guinea-pig ileum contraction by bath application.

| Peptide | Study | | | | | |
	Yajima et al. (1973)	Bury and Mashford (1976)	Oehme et al. (1977)	Yanaihara et al. (1977)	Sandberg and Lee (1979)	
SP	1.0	1.0	1.0	1.0	1.0	
SP$_{2-11}$		0.6	0.7	1.0	1.0	
SP$_{3-11}$		1.6	2.3*	1.0	1.9*	
SP$_{4-11}$	0.5–1	2.1*	1.4	0.4	0.9	
SP$_{5-11}$	2–4*	1.3	1.0	0.7 (1.7)†	0.24–0.50‡	
SP$_{6-11}$	2	1.0	0.5	0.3 (2.0)†	0.29–0.55‡ (0.9)†	
SP$_{7-11}$	0.05	0.002	0.003	0.01	0.000 5	
SP$_{8-11}$	0.02	0.000 2		0.01	<0.000 05	
SP$_{9-11}$		0.000 01		0.01	<0.000 05	

* Peak potencies.
† Numbers in parentheses are for cyclized (pyroglutamyl) N-terminal forms.
‡ Range is quoted due to uncertainty in peptide concentration.

exerts potent biological actions, rather little detailed information is available on the nature of the tissue receptors involved. The considerable earlier literature on the peripheral actions of SP and related tachykinins has been reviewed elsewhere (Lembeck and Zetler, 1962; Bernardi, 1966; Bury and Mashford, 1977a). The general availability of pure preparations of synthetic SP and the development of synthetic peptide analogues, however, have been recent developments, allowing for the first time the systematic study of structure–activity relations. Nevertheless, the absence of specific antagonists for SP receptors, and the lack of a radioligand binding assay for such sites are major impediments to studies of the molecular nature and biological importance of such receptors.

The available information, summarized in this review supports the earlier suggestion that the biological actions of SP and other tachykinins are mediated by the same tissue receptors. The peptides in this group (Table 3.1) share a conserved *C*-terminal amino acid sequence: Phe–X–Gly–Leu–Met–NH_2 which appears to be crucial for biological activity. In several systems the tachykinins show cross-tachyphylaxis, supporting the view that they act on a common receptor mechanism (Bury and Mashford, 1977a) (Tables 3.1 and 3.2).

3.2 ACTIONS ON PERIPHERAL TISSUES

3.2.1 Extravascular smooth muscle

The atropine-resistant contraction of the isolated rabbit jejunum by SP was used by von Euler and Gaddum (1931) in their initial characterization of SP. A number of intestinal smooth muscle preparations have since been shown to respond to SP, including the hen rectal caecum, the rabbit jejunum, the goldfish intestine, and rabbit and human duodenum (for review see Bury and Mashford, 1977a). However, the most extensive and detailed information is available on the guinea-pig ileum.

On this tissue, SP is a very potent stimulant. Rosell *et al.* (1977) determined the EC50 to be 2.5 nM. In this study SP was forty times more potent than acetylcholine and one hundred and sixty times more potent than histamine. The contraction in response to SP involves only the longitudinal muscle, the circular muscle being unaffected. Removal of Auerbach's plexus does not alter the sensitivity to SP, suggesting that the receptors are located directly on the muscle and not on the myenteric plexus neurons (Paton and Zar, 1966). The effect is slowed by histamine or acetylcholine, but accelerated by bradykinin (Bury and Mashford, 1977b). Libonati and Segre (1960) found no differences in the effectiveness of SP when tested at either pH 4.7 and 8.0, but another maximum of activity was later detected between pH 9 and 10 (Walaszek and Dyer, 1966), the range for the isoelectric point of SP. As with other biogenic amine or peptide-induced contractile responses in the ileum, addition of the calcium antagonists Verpamil or 10 mM La^{3+} blocks the effect elicited by SP (Bury and Mashford, 1976). Tetrodotoxin and indomethacin have no effects on the contraction indicating that neither neural inputs nor prostaglandin release are necessary (Bury and Mashford, 1977b).

A number of different studies of the potency relationships of C-terminal fragments of SP have indicated slightly different rank orders of potency (Table 3.2). However, all studies show augmented potency in one or more of the shorter fragments from SP_{3-11} to SP_{6-11}. One variable in assigning the position of maximum activity is that not all groups have used the pyroglutamyl-N-terminal forms of the SP_{5-11} and SP_{6-11} fragments. Work by Yanaihara *et al.* (1977), Kitagawa *et al.* (1978), and Sandberg and Lee (1979) have shown that the cyclized N-terminal forms are more potent than those with free N-terminals in these shorter peptides, possibly because of the enzymatic protection afforded by N-terminal blocking. Oehme *et al.* (1977) made the interesting observation that the preference for SP_{3-11} in normal ileum could be altered to a pattern in which the $SP_{(1 \text{ or } 2)-11}$ and SP_{6-11} fragments were the preferred structures. This was observed in the continued presence of SP-like agonists (eledoisin analogues) and involved both a shift in the dose–response curves and an attenuation of the maximal responses.

A number of analogues of native SP have been synthesized with selective amino acid replacements in an effort to assign functional roles to individual sites. Removal of the C-terminal methionine amide, or its replacement by the free acid eliminates the spasmogenic activity (Yanaihara *et al.*, 1977; Sandberg and Lee, 1979). However, replacement of the C-terminal by norleucine amide (Rietschoten *et al.*, 1975) or leucine amide (Yanaihara *et al.*, 1977) gives analogues with full or nearly full activity. Replacement of glycine at position 9 by D-leucine causes a dramatic loss of activity (Yamaguchi *et al.*, 1979). This may indicate a key structural role for this residue which has been speculated to be the hinge of a flexible C-terminal sequence conserved in all the tachykinins (Folkers *et al.*, 1977). Replacement of phenylalanines at positions 7 and 8 by D-phenylalanine lowers the activity by three orders of magnitude (Yamaguchi *et al.*, 1979). However, substitution by tyrosine in position 8 maintains (Rosell *et al.*, 1977), or even enhances activity (Kitagawa *et al.*, 1978). Replacement of the two phenylalanine residues by isoleucines virtually eliminates activity (Rosell *et al.*, 1977). Manipulations at positions 1 to 5 do not appear to alter the activity to a large degree, suggesting that the 'informational' portion of the molecule for smooth muscle effects is contained in the 6 to 11 sequence. This is in keeping with electrophysiological results (see later), and raises the possibility that SP may be processed to smaller biologically active fragments *in vivo*.

Comparison of these results with earlier work on the related peptides eledoisin and physalaemin supports the general conclusions from the SP work. The stimulant effects of physalaemin on guinea-pig ileum are retained in fragments shortened to the *C*-terminal hexapeptide (Bernardi *et al.*, 1966). Indeed, the octapeptide and hexapeptide are more active than the intact molecule. The five *C*-terminal residues are the minimum required for detectable activity on the ileum (Bernardi *et al.*, 1966). Similar results were reported for eledoisin, with the *C*-terminal octa-, nona- and decapeptides having greater activity than the full sequence (Bernardi *et al.*, 1964). A number of physalaemin or eledoisin analogues containing the fundamental tachykinin sequence of Phe–X–Gly–Leu–Met–NH$_2$ are all highly active (see Bury and Mashford, 1977a, for references). Residue substitution studies on *C*-terminal hexapeptides of physalaemin and eledoisin and hepta- and octapeptides of physalaemin indicate that alteration of phenylalanine 7 or leucine 10 lead to loss of activity (Bury and Mashford, 1977a). The *C*-terminal methionine amide of either peptide can be replaced by neutral amino acids without destroying biological potency, and its replacement by ethionine or alkyl homocysteineamides increases the effectiveness on the ileum (Bernardi *et al.*, 1965).

The *C*-terminal amide function can be replaced by the nitrile, but its removal or oxidation of the methionine amide to the sulphone reduces the activity (Camerino *et al.*, 1963, Sandrin and Boissonnas, 1964). Glycine 9 can be replaced by sarcosine or alanine, but not by phenylalanine (Bernardi *et al.*, 1964). The *C*-terminal pentapeptide of physalaemin is more potent than the corresponding fragment of eledoisin; these pentapeptides differ structurally only at position 8 where an aromatic group (Tyr) occurs in physalaemin (Bury and Mashford, 1977a). Hexapeptides with *N*-terminal basic amino acids (lysine, ornithine, or arginine) are five times less potent than those with neural amino acids (serine, alanine) (Bernardi, 1966; Bernardi *et al.*, 1966). The basic groups, however, do not require their charge since their acetylation does not alter spasmogenic activity (Bernardi *et al.*, 1964, Lübke *et al.*, 1966).

Another approach to defining important regions of the peptides was adopted by Oehme *et al.* (1972), who replaced several positions with the corresponding hydrazino amino acids. Replacement of the *N*-terminal phenylalanine in the *C*-terminal pentapeptide of eledoisin does not affect its activity. The hexa- and octapeptides of eledoisin, more potent than the entire peptide, are reduced to activities equipotent with eledoisin upon substitution of the phenylalanine by the corresponding hydrazino residue. Substitution of hydrazino glycine for glycine in the eledoisin octapeptide attenuates the activity (Oehme *et al.*, 1970). An eledoisin octapeptide in which alpha-azasparagine replaces aspartic acid is several times more active than the octapeptide (Niedrich *et al.*, 1971).

Substitutions by D-amino acids in any portion of the C-terminal pentapeptide destroy activity (Bury and Mashford, 1977a), but substitution of D-lysine for lysine and D-asparagine for asparagine yields active physalaemin analogues (Bernardi, 1966), as does D-lysine substitution in eledoisin (Schröder *et al.*, 1965). None of the D-substituted analogues of eledoisin or physalaemin have any antagonistic potency against eledoisin (Schröder *et al.*, 1965).

Yamaguchi *et al.* (1979) have systematically pursued the search for a specific peptide antagonist by selective D-amino acid substitutions in SP and shorter fragments. One analogue, (D-Phe^7)-SP, has detectable antagonistic activity at 1 µM. Another systematic approach that has been suggested is to explore the effects of lengthening the N-terminal of SP by structurally different amino acids (Bury and Mashford, 1977a).

3.2.2 Cardiovascular effects

The intravenous or intra-arterial injection of SP causes peripheral vasodilation and a fall in blood pressure in all mammalian species tested (for review see Bury and Mashford, 1977a). In some cases, the hypotensive effect is subsequently followed by a hypertensive response. There is no evidence for direct cardiotropic effects of SP.

The activity profiles of SP fragments on venoconstriction and blood flow are shown in Table 3.3. The two responses show similar rank orders of potency, with a peak of activity in the SP_{4-11} segment. SP venoconstriction in the rabbit ear vein shows marked desensitization which also affects

Table 3.3 Cardiovascular potencies of substance P fragments with systemic administration. (Bury and Mashford, 1976).

Peptide	Rabbit venoconstriction	Dog arterial blood flow
SP	1.0	1.0
SP_{2-11}	0.9	0.7
SP_{3-11}	1.1	1.3
SP_{4-11}	1.3	1.6
SP_{5-11}	1.0	1.0
SP_{6-11}	0.5	0.6
SP_{7-11}	0.001	0.04

eledoisin responses, but not those of bradykinin (Bury and Mashford, 1977a). Hypotensive potencies of *C*-terminal fragments of eledoisin and physalaemin follow the pattern of effects on spasmogenic activity, although even the most active fragments were only marginally more potent than the parent peptides (Bernardi, 1966). Traczyk (1977) found that the SP *C*-terminal hexapeptide is equivalent to SP in its potency on the cardiovascular systems of dogs, cats, guinea pigs, and rats. The pyroglutamyl-*N*-terminal form of the hexapeptide is even more potent than SP. SP and physalaemin have a greater relative potency in lowering blood pressure when compared to eledoisin than they do on ileum contraction. This enhancement in cardiovascular potency may depend on the presence of an aromatic residue at position 8 in SP and physalaemin (Bury and Mashford, 1977a).

The rabbit mesenteric vein has recently been proposed as a specific bioassay for SP. It can be made specific by the use of selective inhibitors of acetylcholine, catecholamines, serotonin, and histamine, as well as bradykinin using an antagonist, (des–Arg^9–Leu–OMe^8)-bradykinin, which is specific for this preparation (Bérubé *et al.*, 1978). The effect of SP on the vein appears to be direct and not mediated through other transmitters. The involvement of prostaglandins is ruled out because of the lack of any effect of pre-treatment with indomethacin. Dose–response curves follow mass-action predictions, and indicate an EC50 for SP of 74 nM.

Yanaihara *et al.* (1977) found that (Leu^{11})–SP is 3 per cent and (N^α–Tyr)–SP 30 per cent as active as SP on cat blood pressure. (des–Met^{11})–SP is nearly four orders of magnitude weaker than SP (Table 3.3).

3.2.3 Sialogogue activity

Leeman and Hammerschlag (1967) and Lembeck and Starke (1968) demonstrated the stimulant effects of SP on salivation following injection in anaesthetized rats. This effect is not blocked by atropine, propranolol, or phenoxybenzamine and appears to be a direct one on the glands themselves, not mediated through neural stimulation. This interpretation is supported by subsequent biochemical data showing direct effects of SP on isolated fragments of salivary glands (Rudich and Butcher, 1976; Spearman and Pritchard, 1977; Putney, 1979).

The structure–activity profile for *C*-terminal SP fragments on salivation differs from those for intestinal smooth muscle and hypotension. In two studies (Table 3.4), activity was found to fall off with progressive shortening of the peptide. Thus, unlike the other two responses, saliva production appears to require the entire SP sequence for full activity. The sialogogue response is, furthermore, nearly three orders of magnitude less

Table 3.4 Sialogogic potencies of substance P fragments in the rat with systemic administration.

Peptide	Leeman et al. (1977)	Hanley et al. (1980)
SP	1.0	1.0
SP_{2-11}		0.26
SP_{3-11}		0.16
SP_{4-11}	0.12	0.37
SP_{5-11}	0.15	0.24–0.32†
SP_{6-11}		0.17 (0.4)*
SP_{7-11}		<0.003

* Number in parentheses refers to cyclized (pyroglutamyl) *N*-terminal form.
† Range is quoted due to uncertainty in peptide concentration.

sensitive to systemic doses of SP than the hypotensive activity. However, these conclusions must be viewed with caution inasmuch as the metabolic instability of SP and related peptides in blood may alter their apparent activity on salivary glands. Indeed, Lembeck *et al.* (1978a) used the time course of the salivary response to monitor the rate of SP disappearance from the circulation when SP is administered to different vascular regions (Table 3.4).

3.2.4 Other effects

Mills *et al.* (1974) found that infusion of low doses (1 to 100 ng/min) of SP in the dog renal artery causes diuretic and natriuretic changes accompanied by an increase in kallikrein excretion. Proximal tubular reabsorption of salt and water, unrelated to changes in kidney and individual glomerular filtration rates, plasma flow, or intrarenal hydrostatic pressure, are reduced by intra-arterial SP (Arendshorst *et al.*, 1976). In addition, intrarenal SP suppresses renin release in the presence and absence of diuresis, natriuresis, and vasodilation (Gullner *et al.*, 1979). These studies point to a possible role of circulating SP as a renal regulatory hormone.

Although SP was reported to be a stimulant of afferent nerve endings by Lembeck (1957) and Juan and Lembeck (1974), Stewart *et al.* (1976) found that synthetic SP was not algesic on application to the base of human blisters, and suggested that the original results might be explained by contamination of the SP extracts by kinins. More recent work by Lembeck and Gamse (1977) supports the latter conclusion since neither synthetic nor highly purified extracted SP has detectable algesic activity.

SP, like other hypotensive peptides, can also trigger histamine release from mast cells, but eledoisin has no effect (Johnson and Erdös, 1973). Thus, although mast cell histamine release might be an indirect modulator of some of the effects attributed to SP, the lack of pharmacological specificity in this response makes it unclear as to whether an authentic SP receptor is involved.

3.3 ACTIONS ON NEURONS

3.3.1 Direct central effects

The most extensive studies of the possible transmitter role of SP in the nervous system have been in the spinal cord. A SP-like peptide was isolated by Otsuka *et al.* (1972a) from dorsal roots, and shown to have a motoneuron-depolarizing activity in frog spinal cord. Subsequent testing of synthetic SP established that it has a potent excitatory action on both frog spinal motoneurons (Otsuka *et al.*, 1972b) and on new-born rat motoneurons (Konishi and Otsuka, 1974a). Comparison with the action of bath-applied L-glutamate, another candidate for primary afferent neurotransmission, indicated that SP is two hundred times more potent than glutamate on rat motoneurons (Saito *et al.*, 1975a), although Nicoll (1976, 1978) found SP to be only five times more potent than L-glutamate on frog motoneurons. The effects are not blocked by conditions blocking synaptic transmission (0.5 μM tetrodotoxin, reduced calcium, or 8 mM Mg^{2+}) and thus seem to be direct cellular responses. SP receptors appear to be localized to the somatic dendrites of motoneurons since the isolated ventral roots were unresponsive to SP (Nicoll, 1976). The action of SP differed from that of L-glutamate in its longer latency, longer persistence, and smaller maximum depolarization (Nicoll, 1976). The latter was so small that the motoneurons rarely reached spiking threshold (Nicoll, 1978). Addition of the peptidase inhibitor bacitracin did not increase the magnitude of the depolarization. This, and the fact that SP dose–response curves reached plateaus, suggested that receptors were fully occupied and that SP degradation could not be attenuating the response and inhibiting the depolarization potency (Nicoll, 1978). SP causes a reduction in membrane resistance in frog motoneurons (Nicoll, 1978), unlike observations on mammalian motoneurons (Krnjevic, 1977), and on guinea pig myenteric plexus neurons (Katayama and North, 1978) where SP increased membrane resistance, or on cat dorsal horn neurons where membrane resistance was unchanged (Zieglgänsberger and Tulloch, 1979). Nicoll (1978) suggested that the sub-threshold depolarization induced by SP and its long persistence may act to 'set the level of excitability of motoneurons and thus facilitate transmission through fast conducting, powerful pathways which subserve basic reflex activity'. Consistent with this idea, Krivoy *et al.* (1977) observed that low doses of intravenous SP facilitate postdetonation recovery of motoneuron excitability in decerebrate cats, without an increase in excitatory postsynaptic potentials or detectable depolarizations in one-half of the sampled motoneurons.

Henry *et al.* (1975) applied SP iontophoretically to dorsal horn neurons in cat spinal cord and observed an excitation in approximately half of the units with a 15 to 20 s latency, and a duration of 1 to 2 min. SP also potentiates, and occasionally depresses, responses to L-glutamate. Neurons that respond to thermal cutaneous painful stimuli are selectively excited by SP. Subsequent studies have confirmed the selective excitatory effects of SP on spinal cord neurons that receive nociceptive inputs, leading to the suggestion that SP may be involved in transmisstion of nociceptive information (Henry, 1976; Randic and Miletic, 1977; Anderson *et al.*, 1978). In support of this, stimulation of rat dorsal horn units by intra-arterial administration of the algesic peptide bradykinin identifies a population of responsive units that corresponds with those sensitive to iontophoretic excitation by the SP analogue, eledoisin-related peptide (Roberts and Wright, 1978). Fourteen to twenty-one days after unilateral dorsal root section, ipsilateral spinal cord neurons in the rat respond more intensely to iontophoretic application of eledoisin-related peptide by increased firing rates. This was interpreted as evidence of denervation supersensitivity in the SP receptors (Wright and Roberts, 1978).

SP also depolarizes the intramedullary portion of primary afferent fibres (Nicoll, 1976) and is more potent than L-glutamate in this action. The SP receptor appears to be distributed similarly to the glutamate receptor, since the somata of primary afferents are insensitive to either L-glutamate or SP (Barker *et al.*, 1975a). The prolonged action of SP has led to speculation that it might mediate primary afferent depolarization. Picrotoxin (0.2 mM) fails to block the action of SP on primary afferent terminals (Nicoll, 1976), unlike the picrotoxin-induced inhibition of primary afferent depolarization (Barker *et al.*, 1975b). However, it should be noted that Konishi and Otsuka (1974b) observed two phases of SP action on the ventral root monosynaptic reflex, an initial inhibition and a subsequent facilitation. The initial transient depression could be abolished by picrotoxin (0.2 mM).

SP has been applied by iontophoresis to neurons in the amygdala (Le Gal La Salle and Ben-Ari, 1977), locus coeruleus (Guyenet and Aghajanian, 1977), mesencephalic reticular formation (Davies and Dray, 1976a) substantia nigra (Davies and Dray, 1976b; Walker *et al.*, 1976), cerebral cortex (Phillis and Limacher, 1974; Phillis, 1977), cuneate nucleus (Krnjevic and Morris, 1974), and interpeduncular nucleus (Sastry, 1978). In all cases, excitation was the most frequently observed response, although examples of depression were detected in the s. nigra and cortex.

The onset latencies for excitation induced by SP were shorter in most brain areas than for spinal cord neurons, but were still much longer in all cases than those for iontophoretically applied L-glutamate. However, the slow onset of excitation evoked by iontophoretically applied SP may be due to its very low transport number and delayed release from iontophoretic electrodes; under optimum conditions very rapid (<5 s) excitatory responses can be observed (Guyenet *et al.*, 1979). Several types of interactions between SP and other putative CNS transmitter candidates have been observed. Krnjevic and Morris (1974) found that SP excitation in the cuneate nucleus is antagonized by GABA, and L-glutamate excitation is inhibited by SP. Sastry (1978) observed a synergism between muscarinic acetylcholine responses and SP effects in the interpeduncular nucleus. SP is one of the most potent excitants of cerebral cortical neurons (Phillis, 1977). SP-responsive neurons were all spontaneously active units and no excitatory effects were seen on silent cortical cells (Phillis, 1977).

In guinea-pig myenteric plexus neurons, intracellular recordings show a slow depolarization mediated by an increase in membrane resistance in response to iontophoretic application of SP. The excitation was dose-dependent, and closely resembled an effect elicited by focal stimulation of the ganglion surface (Katayama and North, 1978).

SP co-ordinately affects both pre- and post-synaptic sites in two cholinergic systems. In the Mauthner fibre–giant fibre synapse of the hatchet-fish, 1 to 100 µM SP causes a dose-dependent reduction in post-synaptic potentials and miniature post-synaptic potential amplitudes after 30 to 45 s. In addition, it also causes, at higher concentrations, a reduction in quantal content, suggesting pre-synaptic inhibition. The net result is a persistent (10 to 20 min) depression of synaptic transmission after SP application (Steinacker and Highstein, 1976). Extension of this work to the frog neuromuscular junction revealed that there were two sequential phases of SP action at 1 to 10 µM concentrations. In the first phase, both excitatory post-synaptic potential amplitude and quantal content decline, followed by a recovery within 30 to 40 min and then a 2 to 3 h period of increased synaptic transmission with augmented post-synaptic potential amplitude and increased quantal content (Steinacker, 1977). The initial phase is calcium-responsive since augmentation of the external calcium to twice normal levels abolishes the depression. It is unclear, given the high SP concentrations and the lack of more extensive pharmacology of the responses, whether these effects are receptor-mediated, or non-specific interactions with membrane components. Somatostatin at similar high concentrations induces a non-selective leakage of synaptosomal contents (Nemeth and Cooper, 1979). SP and other peptides may exhibit ionophoric or membrane effects at very high concentrations.

3.3.2 Structure-function

Davies and Dray (1976b) found that the stimulation of neurons in rat substantia nigra by SP is mimicked by eledoisin, and Wright and Roberts (1978) used eledoisin-related peptide interchangeably with SP in excitation of dorsal horn neurons. Guyenet and Aghajanian (1977) observed that eledoisin, physalaemin, and SP were equally effective in exciting rat locus coeruleus neurons, but that activation by SP_{4-11} was more rapid in onset and reversal than that elicited by SP itself.

The most extensive investigation of the structural requirements for responses of neurons in CNS to SP is that of Otsuka *et al.* (1975) and Otsuka and Konishi (1976) (Table 3.5). In both frog and rat spinal motoneurons, the *C*-terminal portion of the molecule, shared by all tachykinins, is essential. The *C*-terminal methionine amide can be replaced with leucine amide with only a slight loss of activity. Interestingly, the rank order of potencies on rat motoneurons shows an enhancement of activity relative to SP in the SP_{5-11} and S_{6-11} fragments. One important difference between the results on frog and rat motoneurons is that the SP_{6-11} fragment is reduced in activity relative to SP on frog motoneurons, but is much more potent than SP on rat motoneurons. This has led to the suggestion that a shorter fragment of SP may be the true endogenous transmitter (Otsuka and Konishi, 1976; Phillis, 1977). It should also be considered that SP may be related to a family of peptide transmitters, and shorter fragments may themselves act as separate transmitters, or be related to other active peptides (Table 3.5).

Table 3.5 Potencies of substance P fragments in motoneuron depolarization by bath application.

Peptide	Rat (Otsuka and Konishi, 1976)	Frog (Otsuka *et al.*, 1975)
SP	1.0	1.0
SP_{2-11}	0.6–0.9	
SP_{3-11}	0.4–1.0	
SP_{4-11}	0.8–1.0	0.075
SP_{5-11}	2–12	
SP_{6-11}	5–12	<0.025
SP_{7-11}	<0.02	<0.006
SP_{8-11}	<0.000 2	<0.000 5
SP_{9-11}	<0.000 08	<0.000 02
des-Met[11]-SP	<0.000 5	

3.3.3 Baclofen as a specific SP antagonist

Baclofen (Lioresal; beta-(4-chlorophenyl)-gamma-aminobutyric acid) is a centrally-acting muscle relaxant (Fox *et al.*, 1978). Saito *et al.* (1975b) reported that it acts as a specific antagonist of SP excitation on rat spinal neurons, blocking both the responses to applied SP and the excitatory post-synaptic potentials produced by dorsal root stimulation. A number of experiments have failed to confirm the claimed specificity of this antagonist action. On cerebral cortical neurons, baclofen antagonizes both SP and acetylcholine-induced excitations to a similar extent, as well as supressing spontaneous activity (Phillis, 1977). Similar experiments on the spinal cord (Davies and Dray, 1976a; Henry and Ben-Ari, 1976; Puil *et al.*, 1976), sympathetic ganglia (Fotherby *et al.*, 1976), and cuneate nucleus (Fox *et al.*, 1978) all point to a non-specific general depressant action, although there may be some preferential action of baclofen on primary afferent responses in the spinal cord (Fox *et al.*, 1978).

3.3.4 Interactions with other CNS receptors

Davies and Dray (1977) suggested that SP may interact with opiate receptors because the excitation of Renshaw cells induced by SP is antagonized by naloxone. However, biochemical experiments have not supported this as 10 μM SP has no effect on the binding of the opiate ligand ^{3}H-dihydromorphine to brain membranes (Terenius, 1976); furthermore, SP is pharmacologically unlike other opiate ligands. There is no evidence for any antagonism by naloxone of SP responses in the spinal cord (Henry, 1978) or locus coeruleus (Guyenet and Aghajanian, 1979).

Henry *et al.* (1975) reported that SP antagonizes the L-glutamate-induced excitation of Renshaw cells, although Nicoll (1976) was unable to confirm this observation. More recently, Vincent and Barker (1979) have shown that SP can depress the excitatory action of L-glutamate on mouse spinal cord neurons in culture, suggesting that SP may exert a modulatory effect on glutamate receptors.

Davies and Dray (1976b) observed cross-tachyphylaxis between GABA and eledoisin during iontophoretic application of these substances to rat striatal neurons. Prolonged exposure to eledoisin caused desensitization not only to its own effects but also a decline in responsiveness to GABA and acetylcholine as well.

Low doses of SP can selectively antagonize the nicotinic receptor activation on Renshaw cells by iontophoretically applied acetylcholine (Belcher and Ryall, 1977; Krnjevic and Lekic, 1977; Ryall and Belcher, 1977). Krnjevic and Lekic (1977) found that SP had no inhibitory effect on stimulation of Renshaw cells through the ventral roots, and suggested that activation of the pathway by root stimulation is sufficiently efficient to mask completely any inhibitory effect of SP. On the other hand, Ryall and Belcher (1977) were able to show an inhibitory effect of SP with submaximal ventral root volleys. SP alone generally has little effect on Renshaw cells, although in some instances, SP induced a transient and rapidly desensitizing excitatory action which was blocked by dihydro-β-erythroidine, suggesting an activation of nicotinic receptors (Belcher and Ryall, 1977). Livett *et al*. (1979) have confirmed the ability of SP to modulate nicotinic receptors using another system. In isolated chromaffin cells from the adrenal medulla, SP caused a dose-dependent reduction (IC50 = 500 nM) in acetylcholine-stimulated ^{3}H-norepinephrine release, an effect mediated by nicotinic receptors.

3.4 BIOCHEMICAL STUDIES

3.4.1 Binding studies

SP is notable among the neurotransmitter candidates in that, although the evidence is stronger for its neurotransmitter role than for other peptides, there have so far been no unequivocal receptor binding studies with radiolabelled derivatives of SP. Three preliminary accounts have appeared and will be considered.

Nakata *et al*. (1978) prepared (^{3}H)–SP by platinum-catalysed tritium gas exposure (Segewa *et al*., 1976) of synthetic SP, and subsequent purification of the reaction products by Sephadex gel chromatography. In early experiments on SP uptake the specific activity of the ^{3}H–SP was 1.31 Ci/mmol, and the biological activity on the guinea-pig ileum was estimated to be 80 per cent that of synthetic SP (Segawa *et al*., 1976, 1977). More recently, the same procedures were reported to yield (^{3}H)–SP with a specific activity of 187 Ci/mmol, and with full contractile activity on the guinea-pig ileum (Nakata *et al*., 1978). The (^{3}H)–SP co-migrated with synthetic SP in thin layer and Sephadex gel chromatographic systems of low resolving power.

The binding of (^{3}H)–SP was studied using crude synaptic membrane preparation from rabbit brain that had been stored at $-30°$ C (Nakata *et al*., 1978). The highest density of specific binding sites, defined by using 'a large excess of unlabelled substance P' for non-specific binding, was in the diencephalon, with low levels in the cortex and hippocampus. Scatchard analysis of the concentration-dependent saturation of specific ^{3}H–SP binding to brain stem membranes indicated a maximum number of binding sites of 95.7 fmol/mg protein and an apparent dissociation constant of 2.74 nM. These values are in reasonable agreement with those found for other putative peptide neurotransmitters (cf. Chapter 5). Fragments of SP

Table 3.6 Comparison of binding antagonism K_is to rat motoneuron depolarization potencies.

Peptide	Nakata *et al.* (1978)	Mayer *et al.* (1979)	Otsuka and Konishi (1976)
SP	0.003 17 µM	0.17 µM	1.0
SP_{2-11}		2.8 µM	0.6–0.9
SP_{3-11}	2.8 µM	7.8 µM	0.4–1.0
SP_{4-11}	0.34 µM	8.8 µM	0.8–1.0
SP_{5-11}	0.056 µM		2–12
SP_{6-11}	0.001 3 µM		5–12
SP_{7-11}	0.48 µM		<0.02
SP_{8-11}			<0.000 2
SP_{9-11}			<0.000 08
Eledoisin	5.9 µM	No antagonism	
Physalaemin	>10 µM	Enhanced binding of $^{125}I\text{-}Tyr^8\text{-}SP$	

antagonised (^3H)–SP binding in a rank order of potencies similar to their potencies in depolarizing rat motoneurons (Table 3.6). However, Otsuka and Konishi (1976) found maximum potency in the hexapeptide C-terminal fragment, whereas Nakata *et al.* (1978) found maximum potency in the heptapeptide fragment. Physalaemin and eleoisin were only weakly active (micromolar concentrations) in antagonizing the binding of (^3H)–SP, although they are more effective than SP in depolarizing frog spinal motoneurons (Otsuka *et al.*, 1975) (Table 3.6).

An unusual feature of the assay procedure used by Nakata *et al.* (1978) was that incubations with (^3H)–SP were conducted for only 1 min at 0° C. These conditions fall far short of these needed to attain equilibrium for the binding of other peptides to brain membranes (cf. Chapter 5). In the absence of kinetic data, the issue cannot be resolved, but it should be noted that if the incubations did not allow equilibrium to be established, the results cannot be compared quantitatively with those of other studies, and the SP fragment competition results may be unreliable.

Lembeck *et al.* (1978b) explored a different approach to SP binding studies. Extraction of brain homogenates by organic solvents at neutral pH to produce a total lipid extract (2:1 vol/vol chloroform:methanol) was shown to extract most of the biologically active SP. On chromatographic analysis of the extract on Sephadex LH-20 the SP biological activity migrated with phospholipids. Subsequent analysis of the lipid content of these fractions revealed a high content of acidic phospholipids, particularly phosphatidyl serine. The pH dependence of phosphatidyl serine adsorption of synthetic SP closely resembled the adsorption behaviour of the total lipid extract for endogenous SP. Accordingly, it was suggested that phosphatidyl serine might represent a physiologically important storage site for SP, and might also participate in SP receptor function.

The solvent-extraction protocol was subsequently used to investigate the binding of (^{125}I–Tyr)–SP to a 'synaptic vesicle' subcellular fraction from rat brain (Mayer *et al.*, 1979). The Tyr^8 analogue of SP was radioiodinated with ^{125}I and purified to the monoiodinated species by sulphopropyl–Sephadex chromatography, giving a final product with a 0.6 Ci/mmol specific activity. The specific binding of (^{125}I–Tyr^8)–SP to a synaptic vesicle preparation indicated the presence of a single population of sites with an apparent K_d of 0.32 (equilibrium determination) or 0.1 nM (kinetic determination), and a total binding capacity of 800 fmol/mg protein. These values do not agree with those of Nakata *et al.* (1978) and support the interpretation that this procedure is examining a different SP binding site from that described by Nakata *et al.* (1978). In agreement with this proposition, Saria *et al.* (1978) have shown that (^{125}I–Tyr^8)–SP exhibits very different binding properties to a synaptic plasma membrane fraction from rat brain, indicating the presence of two sites (K_d = 0.26 and 1.9 nM) with lower binding capacities (9 and 90 fmol/mg protein, respectively) than in the synaptic vesicle fraction. Furthermore, the regional distribution of synaptic vesicle binding sites in rat brain had the rank order: medulla > midbrain > hypothalamus > striatum > cortex > cerebellum, whereas the regional distribution of synaptic plasma membrane binding sites was: striatum > medulla, midbrain, cortex, cerebellum > hypothalamus. The distribution of the synaptic vesicle binding sites is similar to the distribution of endogenous SP (Cuello *et al.*, 1978). (^{125}I–Tyr^8)–SP binding to the synaptic vesicle fraction was inhibited by shorter *C*-terminal fragments of SP (Table 3.6) and by SP itself, but surprisingly not by Tyr^8–SP (Mayer *et al.*, 1979), leading the authors to the somewhat unlikely proposal that 'adding the I atom to the phenolic group of Tyr^8 seems to restore the structure and binding affinity'. Moreover, SP$_{3-11}$ and SP$_{4-11}$ and physalaemin actually enhanced specific binding of ^{125}I–Tyr^8 over certain concentration ranges. The unusual pharmacological features of this site have no parallel from other studies, and it does not appear to correspond to a receptor mediating the biological actions of SP.

Mayer and Saria (1979) further reported that the binding of (^{125}I–Tyr^8)–SP to synaptic vesicle fractions was antagonized by millimolar concentrations of Ca^{2+} and Mg^{2+}, and was abolished by pre-treatment of the vesicle fraction with trypsin or with phospholipases A$_2$, C or D.

The interpretation of the SP binding results reported by this group is unclear, because the lipid extraction methodology employed will only measure SP interactions with lipid components. Lipids have been shown to sequester opiates (Loh *et al.*, 1974), nicotinic ligands (Cho *et al.*, 1978), and aromatic amines (Hoss and Smiley, 1977), but these interactions have not been shown under physiological conditions. Thus, to impute a physiological significance to *in vitro* interactions of this type must remain speculative.

Wheeler *et al.* (1979) have reported encouraging preliminary findings on the binding of ^{125}I–physalaemin to dispersed parotid acinar cells, which may reflect SP receptor binding. They found that labelled physalaemin binding is rapid ($t^{1/2} < 2$ min) and saturable with a K_d of 1.4 nM and maximum binding sites of 1.67 fmol/mg protein, or about 215 sites per cell. The potencies of four peptides, SP, physalaemin, (Tyr^8)–SP and SP$_{5-11}$ as inhibitors of ^{125}I–physalaemin binding correlate well ($r = 0.96$) with the potencies of these substances in stimulating ^{86}Rb release from parotid slices. These authors also reported that (^{125}I–Tyr^8)–SP could not be used as an effective receptor ligand in this preparation.

See note added in proof, p. 103.

3.4.2 Receptor-coupled responses

In many receptor systems the characteristics of the receptor can be studied by measurements of biochemical changes that are triggered by receptor occupancy. For example, the structural requirements and localization of catecholamine receptors in CNS have been investigated by measurements of the receptor-coupled stimulation of cyclic AMP production (Iversen, 1977).

SP has been reported to stimulate cAMP accumulation in both human (Duffy *et al.*, 1975) and rat brain (Duffy and Powell, 1975) particulate fractions. Half-maximal stimulation was observed with 180 nM SP in the rat brain and was inhibited by Ca^{2+} (Duffy and Powell, 1975). There was no correlation between the levels of endogenous SP in different brain regions and the magnitude of the cAMP response (Duffy *et al.*, 1975). However, a re-investigation failed to show any change in cAMP formation either in tissue slices or homogenates from various regions of rat brain, using up to 10 µM SP (Quik *et al.*, 1978). Very high concentrations (100 µM) of SP were reported to produce a transient rise in cAMP content in cultured neuroblastoma cells and in intact dorsal root ganglia (Narumi and Fujita, 1978). The characteristics of the tissue response were not investigated in detail, but the effect of SP was similar to that elicited by mouse nerve growth factor. Both agents cause a three-fold increase in the basal levels of cAMP within 10 min, followed by a decline to basal levels by 30 min. Both SP and nerve growth factor stimulate neurite extension during the 24 h period following their addition. Because the direct addition of dibutyryl-cAMP also stimulates neurite extension it was postulated that the effects of both SP and nerve growth factor may be mediated by the transient change in cyclic nucleotide content.

In the same way that the pineal gland has been used as a convenient model for studies of β-adrenoceptors (Axelrod, 1974), the rat parotid gland represents an accessible system for SP receptor studies. Rudich and Butcher (1976) found that in slices of rat parotid gland SP and eledoisin induced rapid concentration- and calcium-dependent increases in K^+ efflux and amylase release. Neither effect was blocked by α- or β-adrenoceptor antagonists or by muscarinic antagonists. Neither eledoisin nor SP caused any change in basal cAMP or cGMP levels. It was suggested that the actions of SP in the parotid gland were mediated by Ca^{2+}. However, a recent study of the response of the rat submandibular gland to physalaemin and eledoisin-related peptide (Spearman and Pritchard, 1977) showed that although the physalaemin-induced K^+ efflux was calcium-dependent, that caused by the eledoisin-related peptide was not. Jones and Michell (1978) observed that 100 nM SP stimulates phosphatidyl inositol turnover in rat parotid gland fragments in a calcium-independent manner. This was interpreted as evidence in favour of the hypothetical general mechanism for receptor coupling to Ca^{2+} fluxes through the intermediate of phosphatidyl inositol membrane lipids (Michell, 1975). Marier *et al.* (1978) have shown that SP triggers the same sequence of events in parotid gland slices as do muscarinic and α-adrenoceptor agonists. Using ^{86}Rb loading of slices to study potassium movements, it was observed that SP stimulated a biphasic release of ^{86}Rb with an initial transient calcium-independent phase and a subsequent sustained calcium-dependent phase. Calcium may, therefore, function as a 'second messenger' between receptor occupancy and potassium fluxes in this tissue. Intriguingly, SP-induced ^{86}Rb efflux was different from that induced by the other two agonist types in that it was not inhibited by the local anaesthetics tetracaine and procaine. This may indicate that the coupling mechanism between SP receptors and ion channel activation is qualitatively unlike that for muscarinic or α-adrenoceptors.

3.4.3 Modulation of neurotransmitter release and metabolism

Activation of SP receptors in CNS may lead to changes in neurotransmitter function and from such indirect effects, inferences can possibly be made about the structural requirements of the SP receptors.

The existence of pre-synaptic receptors which modulate the spontaneous and stimulus-evoked release of neurotransmitters is well established (Langer, 1977). Experiments on the modulation of dopamine (DA), serotonin (5-HT), and gamma-aminobutyric acid (GABA) release from slices of rat substantia nigra and corpus striatum show that SP has no effects in concentrations up to 10 μM on the uptake or spontaneous release of these neurotransmitters, but it slightly enhances K^+-induced DA and 5-HT release in the striatum (Starr, 1978). Reubi *et al.* (1978) investigated the release of 5-HT from rat nigral slices *in vitro* and found it to be stimulated by 50 μM SP or eledoisin. The effect of SP appears to be indirect, since it can be blocked by the dopaminergic antagonist alpha-flupenthixol. SP also stimulates the spontaneous release of ^{3}H-dopamine from nigral slices. It was proposed that SP stimulates nigral dopamine neurons which then release dopamine onto 5-HT terminals, in turn releasing 5-HT upon dopaminergic stimulation. Silbergeld and Walters (1979) reported that the uptake and release of ^{3}H-dopamine by striatal synaptosomes are inhibited in a dose-dependent manner by SP in concentrations above 1 nM and that nigral ^{3}H-dopamine uptake and release are increased by SP in concentrations above 10 nM. SP also causes a dose-dependent stimulation of the spontaneous release of immunoreactive somatostatin from hypothalamic slices (Sheppard *et al.*, 1979). This agrees with an earlier study in which intraventricular SP was found to cause a reduction in circulating growth hormone levels, an effect which could be prevented by somatostatin antiserum (Chihara *et al.*, 1978).

Magnusson *et al.* (1976) and Carlsson *et al.* (1978) studied the effects of SP on central monoaminergic neurons by measuring the accumulation of the dopamine and 5-HT precursors dihydroxyphenylalanine (DOPA) and 5-hydroxytryptophan (5-HTP) after inhibition of their enzymatic decarboxylation. An enhancement of catecholamine synthesis was seen with intraventricular doses of SP of more than 20 μg/rat, and of 5-HT synthesis with doses between 6 and 13 μg/rat. In the presence of inhibitors of monoamine synthesis, SP also accelerated the breakdown of DA, NA and 5-HT. This was interpreted as a consequence of increased impulse traffic in monoamine neurons after excitation by SP. Further investigation of these effects showed that they were most pronounced in the NA-rich areas (diencephalon, hemispheres, and lower brainstem) than in DA-rich areas (limbic forebrain and corpus striatum) (Carlsson *et al.*, 1978). The SP-induced increases in DOPA formation were blocked by systemic administration of naloxone. The structural requirements for the effects were investigated using analogues and fragments of SP (Carlsson *et al.*, 1978) (Table 3.7). (Des–Met^{11})–SP and (Ile^7)–SP were both inactive, implicating the requirement for the *C*-terminal and Phe^7 integrity. The most potent peptides were the analogues (D-Leu^8, D-Phe^9)–SP, (D-Phe^7, D-Phe^8)–SP$_{5-11}$, and (Lys^5, D-Leu^8, D-Phe^9)–SP$_{5-11}$. Reduction of the SP *N*-terminal chain length and D-amino acid substitutions in positions 7 and 8 produced (D-Phe^7, D-Phe^8)–SP$_{5-11}$, the most potent and persistent analogue

Table 3.7 Effects of substance P and synthetic analogues on the formation of DOPA and 5-HTP, and on gross behaviour in rats using intraventricular injection.

Peptide	Dose range (μg/rat)	Effects on		Gross behaviour
		DOPA	5-HTP	
Substance P (SP)	50–120	+	0	+ Rotation
[Ile^7]-SP	50	0	0	(+)
[Des-Met^{11}]-SP	50	0	0	0
[D-Leu^8, D-Phe^9]-SP	50	++	0	++ Rotation
[D-Phe^7, D-Phe^8]-SP	25	++	0	++ Rotation
[Lys^5, D-Leu^8, D-Phe^9]-SP$_{5-11}$	12.5–20	++	+	++ Rotation
[Gly$^{6,7 \text{ or } 8}$]-SP$_{5-11}$	50	+	0	+
SP$_{5-11}$	50	+	0	++ Rotation
[Gly$^{10 \text{ or } 11}$]-SP$_{5-11}$	50	0	0	(+)

Only dominating feature of behavioural pattern is indicated. + and − indicate increased and decreased motor activity, respectively, 0 indicates no change in motor activity, ± periods of increase and decrease. Number of symbols indicate degree of change. Symbol in parenthesis: slight or inconsistent change (Carlsson *et al.*, 1978)

on monoamine turnover. One analogue, (Lys^5, D-Leu^8, D-Phe^9)–SP$_{5-11}$ was the only one which was more potent only on 5-HTP accumulation. Gly^{6,7,8,9} substitution in SP$_{5-11}$ did not alter activity on monoamine turnover relative to native SP, but replacement by Gly in positions 10 and 11 produced inactive analogues.

Cheramy *et al.* (1977) infused 10 nM SP into cat substantia nigra with a push-pull cannula, and found a stimulation of ^{3}H-dopamine synthesis in the ipsilateral caudate nucleus. This was confirmed by Waldmeier *et al.* (1978) who showed a dose-dependent increase in the dopamine metabolites homovanillic acid and 3,4-dihydroxyphenylacetic acid in rat striatum after nigral SP administration; however, much higher SP concentrations were required than in the earlier study. Starr *et al.* (1978) also observed accelerated DA turnover in the rat striatum after peripheral injections of SP, but 5-HT turnover was reduced. Cheramy *et al.* (1978) found that intranigral injection of SP antibodies produced a reduction in ipsilateral striatal ^{3}H-dopamine release and an increase in nigral dendritic release of ^{3}H-dopamine. Michelot *et al.* (1979) reported complementary observations that unilateral nigral infusion of SP or SP$_{4-11}$ increased the spontaneous ^{3}H-dopamine release from the ipsilateral caudate nucleus, and reduced ipsilateral nigral release of ^{3}H-dopamine.

3.5 BEHAVIOURAL RESPONSES TO SP

3.5.1 Effects on activity

The results of early attempts to investigate the central actions of SP are difficult to interpret because of the uncertain purity of the SP preparations used (see Haefely and Hürlimann, 1962). Stern and Hukovic (1960), for instance, found that partially purified preparations of SP elicited markedly different effects from those produced by the crude SP extracts frequently used in earlier studies. Nevertheless, the conclusion reached by Stern and Dobric (1957) that SP has behavioural depressant properties, described by them as 'physiological tranquillizer' appears to remain valid. Using synthetic SP, given systemically by intramuscular injection in the mouse, Stern and Hadzovic (1973) and Stern *et al.* (1974) confirmed the behavioural depressant effects of the peptide, and found that systemically administered SP is able to penetrate into the brain. They reported that the biologically active SP content of mouse brain is significantly increased (approximately doubled) 15 min after i.m. injection of synthetic SP (0.5 mg/kg), although this increase in brain SP is transient and is no longer apparent 40 min after SP injection. Confirmation of the behavioural depressant effects of systemically administered SP has also been reported by Stewart *et al.* (1976) and by Starr *et al.* (1978). The latter authors found that a very small dose of SP (5 µg/animal) administered subcutaneously or intraperitoneally inhibits spontaneous or amphetamine-induced motor activity in mice, with the effect being most marked 30 to 40 min after SP injection. SP also inhibits exploratory behaviour, assessed by a hole board apparatus. In all of these studies the animals were tranquilized rather than sedated, since they could easily be aroused when handled. A marked decrease in spontaneous motor activity, and a concomitant increase in grooming behaviour was observed by Katz (1979) in mice after direct administration of synthetic SP into the lateral ventricles (12.5 – 100 µg). Neither the decreased locomotor activity nor the increased grooming elicited by SP were antagonized by naloxone. Interestingly, Katz (1979) observed that a minority (approximately 1/10) of the animals tested show a paradoxical response with increased motor activity and a Straub tail response (i.e. tail elevation) typical of the running response elicited by opiates in mice. This behavioural activation is seen especially after high doses of SP (>25 µg). This may explain why Carlsson *et al.* (1977) observed a general excitatory response in rats following the injection of relatively large doses of SP and SP analogues into the lateral ventricles (50 to 120 µg/animal). They described a response which consists initially of rotation towards the side of the injection, followed by a longer period of hyperactivity. The results obtained with various synthetic analogues of SP are summarized in Table 3.7. In contrast to the effects on catecholamine turnover, these excitatory responses to SP are *not* antagonized by naloxone. The differences in the responses to SP seen in rats and mice, however, may be related to species differences rather than to the dose of peptide administered. Rondeau *et al.* (1978) administered synthetic SP intraventricularly to rats using a wide range of doses (0.7 to 80.0 μg) and found that motor activity is significantly increased following doses of 0.3 and 1.25 μg; higher doses (40 and 80 μg) cause immobility and rigidity. Microinjection of SP into the medial forebrain bundle region of rat brain at large doses (60 to 120 μg) causes a significant suppression of self-stimulation behaviour elicited by stimulating electrodes in the same site (Goldstein and Malick, 1977) (Table 3.7).

On the other hand, stimulation of locomotor activity has been observed following the direct injection of SP into discrete areas of rat brain. Thus, unilateral injections of SP into the substantia nigra of rat brain cause the animals to turn in a direction contralateral to the injection site (Olpe and Koella, 1977; James and Starr, 1977). Olpe and Koella (1977) found that the turning behaviour is consistently in this direction and requires doses of 2.5 to 10 μg. The eledoisin-related peptide injected at similar doses elicits the same response. James and Starr (1979), however, reported that both contralateral and ipsilateral turning can be elicited by SP (1 to 10 μg), the direction of turning being dependent on the precise injection site within the substantia nigra. Kelley and Iversen (1978) found that bilateral injections of SP (3 μg on each side) in the substantia nigra of rat brain cause increased locomotor activity and stereotyped grooming behaviour, similar to that seen after activation of the nigrostriatal dopamine system by amphetamine. The stimulant effects of SP in behaviour when administered into this region of brain are consistent with biochemical and physiological observations that microinjections of SP into substantia nigra activate the nigral dopamine neurons (Davies and Dray, 1976b; Chéramy *et al.*, 1977; Waldmeier *et al.*, 1978; James and Starr, 1979). Activation of dopamine neurons in the ventral tegmental area (the A10 group) may also explain the excitatory effects on behaviour after bilateral injections of SP into this brain area (Iversen *et al.*, 1978; Stinus *et al.*, 1978; Kelley *et al.*, 1979). In this case further support for the hypothesis that the behavioural excitation is mediated by dopaminergic pathways was provided by the finding that the hyperactivity response to SP can be antagonized by the potent dopamine antagonist fluphenazine and is no longer seen in animals treated with 6-hydroxydopamine to destroy the dopamine neurons of the A10 system (Kelley *et al.*, 1979). Although the behavioural activation seen after intracerebral injections of SP persists for only 30 to 60 min, a prolonged effect on the dopamine neurons appears to occur, as animals remain hypersensitive to the excitant effects of d-amphetamine for up to 24 h after SP injection (Iversen *et al.*, 1978).

Thus, the nature of the behavioural responses to SP is highly dependent on the species and dose used and the route and site of administration. Low doses of peptide given intraventricularly or systemically appear to have a predominantly depressant effect, whereas larger doses given intraventricularly or into dopamine-rich areas of brain have excitatory effects followed by persistent changes in the excitability of CNS dopaminergic mechanisms.

3.5.2 Effects on pain

Similar considerations may explain the apparently contradictory results obtained in experiments designed to test the analgesic properties of SP. The evidence which suggests that SP in primary sensory fibres may be associated with the transmission of pain might suggest that the direct administration of SP should lower pain thresholds, or cause hyperalgesia, and indeed such a response has been reported after administration of relatively large doses of SP systemically (1 to 2 mg/kg) (Zetler, 1956; Juan and Lembeck, 1974) or intraventricularly (0.5 to 1.0 µg) (Frederickson *et al.*, 1978). Zetler (1956), Stern and Hadzovic (1973) and Stern *et al.* (1974) also reported that SP significantly antagonized the analgesic effects of morphine in animals. On the other hand, several more recent reports suggest that SP at much lower doses possesses significant analgesic properties, mediated by a naloxone-sensitive mechanism. Thus, Stewart *et al.* (1976) found that SP administered intracerebrally (2 ng) or i.p. (1 µg) had a prolonged analgesic effect in mice, measured by the hot plate test, with a latency of onset of 30 to 60 min. Starr *et al.* (1978) confirmed these observations, using doses of 1 or 5 µg systemically in mice. Potent and long-lasting analgesia, assessed by the tail flick test, was also reported following injections of SP (0.3 to 10.0 µg) into the midbrain periaqueductal grey region of rat brain (Malick and Goldstein, 1978). In each case the analgesic effects of SP can be completely or partially reversed by naloxone. The apparently paradoxical results on the hyperalgesic versus analgesic actions of SP are perhaps best explained by the results reported by Frederickson *et al.* (1978). They found that SP produced naloxone-reversible analgesia in mice when very small doses (1 to 5 ng) were injected intraventricularly. Higher doses of SP produced hyperalgesia when given with naloxone, and continued to cause analgesia when combined with baclofen. The authors suggest that SP may have a dual action, releasing endorphins at low doses and directly exciting neuronal activity in nociceptive pathways at higher doses. This would imply that baclofen can effectively antagonize the latter responses, and indeed Wilson and Yaksh (1978) found that baclofen produces a potent naloxone-insensitive anti-nociceptive effect when administered intrathecally into the lumbar subarachnoid space of the spinal cord in conscious rats.

The effect is seen at doses as low as 10 to 100 ng, and is specific for the pharmacologically active (−) enantiomer of the drug. These results are of considerable pharmacological interest, since they suggest the possibility of developing novel non-opiate analgesic drugs from a better understanding of SP mechanisms.

3.5.3 Drinking behaviour

Highly specific behavioural effects of SP on drinking have been observed, with puzzling species differences. Thus, in the pigeon, direct intracranial injections of SP and eledoisin causes the animals to drink water (Evered *et al.*, 1977). The response is similar to that elicited by the potent dipsogen angiotensin II, and with higher doses of eledoisin (1 nmol) the animals drink more than they normally would during an entire day within a period of less than 5 min. Eledoisin is approximately 100 times more potent than SP in this test, and is only 10 times less potent than angiotensin II, the effective dose range for eledoisin being between 10 and 1000 ng. In the rat, however, SP and related peptides have the opposite effect, and act as potent antidipsogens (De Caro *et al.*, 1977, 1978a,b). Intracranial injections of eledoisin, physalaemin and SP in rats strongly inhibit the drinking responses normally elicited by antiotensin II, carbachol, water deprivation or salt loading. The most potent effects are seen with SP, and particularly when water intake is induced by injections of angiotensin II into the preoptic area. In these experiments drinking is inhibited by doses of SP as low as 1 ng. These results suggest that in the rat, in contrast to the pigeon, SP acts as a thirst inhibitor, although angiotensin II is a potent dipsogen in both species, and in all other vertebrates tested. Whatever the explanation of these species differences, the effects of SP on drinking behaviour seems to offer a sensitive and specific model for assessing a central action of SP and related peptides.

3.6 CONCLUSIONS

The tissue receptors for SP share similarities with those responsible for mediating the actions of other biologically active peptides. The actions of SP are relatively slow and persistent by comparison with those of most conventional amine or amino acid neurotransmitters, and responses are often elicited by very low (nanomolar) concentrations of peptide, suggesting that the receptors possess a high-affinity recogition site. The nature of the cellular events triggered by SP receptor occupation remains unclear, but it is possible that changes in phosphatidyl inositol turnover and mobilization of cellular calcium may be related key events. Unlike some other biologically active peptides, the actions of SP do not appear to be coupled to cyclic nucleotide mechanisms.

SP receptors occur in a number of clearly defined cellular sites. In the CNS these include both pre- and post-synaptic localizations, and furthermore SP in some situations may interact with and modulate the function of receptors for other neurotransmitters, notably the nicotonic acetylcholine receptor in CNS. It is not yet clear whether more than one sub-type of SP receptor exists in mammalian tissues. The spasmogenic, hypotensive and neural responses show similar structure-activity profiles for SP, *C*-terminal fragments of SP and other SP analogues. On the other hand the sialogogue activity of SP differs from the other responses in that the entire sequence of SP appears to be required for full biological activity. This might suggest that SP receptors in salivary gland tissue are of a different category from those in other non-neural and neural tissues, although this conclusion may be spurious since the apparent sialogogue potencies of SP and its analogues may be determined more by their relative metabolic stabilities than by true receptor potencies.

The conclusions from existing data on structure–activity relations can only be tentative at this stage. The *C*-terminal pentapeptide sequence is unequivocally required for biological activity. Only limited modifications in this sequence are possible without loss of activity. In general, for chemical modifications in this sequence to be acceptable, they must preserve the chemical and steric character of the residue replaced. It is tempting to speculate that a particular conformation of the *C*-terminal residues may be crucial for receptor recognition. It is perhaps surprising that the strongly basic *N*-terminal residues of SP, which contribute prominently to the physico-chemical properties of the intact peptide, do not appear to be essential for biological activity on most tissues. It may be that the *N*-terminal portion of the molecule is important in the transport and storage of the hydrophobic *C*-terminal informational sequence.

The fact that smaller hydrophobic peptide fragments of SP retain full biological activity may be a useful feature in the future design of centrally acting drugs based on the SP molecule, since such fragments may be expected to penetrate into CNS after systemic administration. An important problem however, will be to design peptide analogues of SP or of its *C*-terminal that are resistant to metabolic degradation. In order to achieve this more information will be needed on the physiologically important sites in the molecule for such metabolic inactivation. In principle, however, the development of stable SP analogues that might possess CNS activity seems technically possible. It is difficult to predict what the pharmacological profile of such compounds would be, although an obvious area of interest is the possibility that novel analgesics or tranquillizers might emerge from such compounds.

Rapid progress in the assessment of SP analogues would clearly be achieved more easily if a specific radioligand receptor binding assay were available, and this seems likely to be accomplished in the near future. Another important need is for the development of specific antagonists for the receptor actions of SP. By analogy with previous work on neurotransmitters, the availability of such antagonists is likely to play a vital role in defining the precise functions of SP as a putative peptide neurotransmitter in the nervous system.

Despite these obvious deficiencies, studies of SP receptor mechanisms remain further advanced than those for most other putative neuropeptide transmitters, with the exception of the endorphins. The wealth of information available on the actions of SP on simple peripheral test systems should prove valuable in future studies of its role and receptor actions in CNS.

REFERENCES

Anderson, R.K., Lund, J.P. and Puil, E. (1978), *Can. J. Physiol. Pharmac.*, **56**, 216–222.

Arendshorst, W.J., Cook, M.A. and Mills, I.H. (1976), *Am. J. Physiol.*, **230**, 1662–1667.

Axelrod, J. (1974), *Science*, **184**, 1341–1348.

Barker, J.L., Nicoll, R. and Padjen, A. (1975a), *J. Physiol.*, **245**, 521–536.

Barker, J.L., Nicoll, R. and Padjen, A. (1975b), *J. Physiol.*, **245**, 537–548.

Belcher, G. and Ryall, R.W. (1977), *J. Physiol.*, **272**, 105–119.

Bernardi, L. (1966), *Hypotensive Peptides* (Erdös, E., Back, N., Sicuteri, F. and Wilde, A., eds), Springer-Verlag, New York, pp. 86–92.

Bernardi, L., Bosisio, G., Chillemi, F., de Caro, G., de Castiglione, R., Erspamer, V., Glaesser, A. and Goffredo, O. (1964), *Experientia*, **20**, 306–309.

Bernardi, L., Bosisio, G., Chillemi, F., de Caro, G., de Castiglione, R., Erspamer, V., Glaesser, A. and Goffredo, O. (1965), *Experientia*, **21**, 695–697.

Bernardi, L., Bosisio, G., Chillemi, F., de Caro, G., de Castiglione, R., Erspamer, V. and Goffredo, O. (1966), *Experientia*, **22**, 29–31.

Bérubé, A., Marceau, F., Drouin, J.N., Rioux, F. and Regoli, D. (1978), *Can. J. Physiol. Pharmac.*, **56**, 603–609.

Bury, R.W. and Mashford, M.L. (1976), *J. med. Chem.*, **19**, 854–856.

Bury, R.W. and Mashford, M.L. (1977a), *Aust. J. exp. Biol. med. Sci.*, **55**, 671–735.

Bury, R.W. and Mashford, M.L. (1977b), *Clin. exp. Pharmac. Physiol.*, **4**, 453–461.

Camerino, B., de Caro, G., Boissonas, R., Sandrin, E. and Stürmer, E. (1963), *Experientia*, **19**, 339–342.

Carlsson, A., Garcia-Sevilla, J.A. and Magnusson, T. (1979), *Central Regulation of the Endocrine System* (Fuxe, K., Hökfelt, T. and Luft, R., eds), Plenum Press, New York.

Carlsson, A., Magnusson, T., Fisher, G.H., Chang, D. and Folkers, K. (1977), in

Substance P, ed. by von Euler, U.S. and Pernow, B., Raven Press, New York, 201–205.

Chang, M.M. and Leeman, S. (1970), *J. biol. Chem.*, **245**, 4784–4790.

Chang, M.M., Leeman, S. and Niall, H.D. (1971), *Nature New Biol.*, **232**, 86–87.

Chéramy, A., Nieoullon, A., Michelot, R. and Glowinski, J. (1977), *Neurosci. Lett.*, **4**, 105–109.

Chéramy, A., Michelot, R., Leviel, V., Nieoullon, A., Glowinski, J. and Kerdelhue, B. (1978), *Brain Res.*, **155**, 404–408.

Chihara, K., Arimura, A., Coy, D.H. and Schally, A. (1978), *Endocrinol.*, **102**, 281–290.

Cho, T.M., Cho, J.S. and Loh, H.H. (1978), *Proc. natn. Acad, Sci. USA*, **75**, 784–788.

Cuello, A.C., Emson, P., Del Fiacco, M., Gale, J., Iversen, L.L., Jessell, T.M., Kanazawa, I., Paxinos, G. and Quik, M. (1978), *Centrally Acting Peptides* (Hughes, J., ed), pp. 135–156.

Davies, J. and Dray, A. (1976a), *Brain Res.*, **107**, 623–627.

Davies, J. and Dray, A. (1976b), *Nature*, **262**, 606–607.

Davies, J. and Dray, A. (1977), *Nature*, **268**, 351–352.

De Caro, G., Massi, M. and Micossi, L.G. (1978a), *J. Physiol.*, **279**, 133–140.

De Caro, G., Massi, M., Micossi, L.G. and Venturi, F. (1978b), *Neuropharmac.*, **17**, 925–929.

De Caro, G., Micossi, L.G. and Piccinin, G. (1977), *Pharmac. Res. Commun.*, **9**, 489–500.

Duffy, M.J. and Powell, D. (1975), *Biochim. Biophys. Acta.*, **385**, 275–280.

Duffy, M.J., Wong, J. and Powell, D. (1975), *Neuropharmac.*, **14**, 615–618.

Erspamer, V. and Anastasi, A. (1966), *Hypotensive Peptides* (Erdös, R.G., Back, N., Sicuteri, F. and Wilde, A., eds), Springer-Verlag, Berlin, pp. 63–75.

Euler, U.S. von, and Gaddum, J.H. (1931), *J. Physiol.*, **72**, 74.

Euler, U.S. von, and Pernow, B. (1977), *Substance P*. Raven Press, New York.

Evered, M.D., Fitzsimons, J.T. and De Caro, G. (1977), *Nature*, **268**, 332–333.

Fisher, G.H., Folkers, K., Pernow, B. and Bowers, C.Y. (1976), *J. med. Chem.*, **19**, 325–328.

Folkers, K., Chang, D., Yamaguchi, I., Wan, Y.-P., Rackur, G. and Fisher, G. (1977), *Substance P*. (von Euler, U.S. and Pernow, B., eds), Raven Press, New York, pp. 19–26.

Fotherby, K.J., Morrish, N.J. and Ryall, R.W. (1976), *Brain Res.*, **113**, 210–213.

Fox, S., Krnjevic, K., Morris, M.E., Puil, E. and Werman, R. (1978), *Neurosci.*, **3**, 495–515.

Frederickson, R.C.A., Burgis, V., Harrell, C.E. and Edwards, J.D. (1978), *Science*, **199**, 1359–1362.

Goldstein, J.M. and Malick, J.B. (1977), *Pharmac. Biochem. Behav.*, **7**, 475–478.

Gullner, H.-G., Campbell, W.B. and Pettinger, W.A. (1979), *Life Sci.*, **24**, 237–246.

Guyenet, P.G. and Aghajanian, G.K. (1977), *Brain Res.*, **136**, 178–184.

Guyenet, P.G. and Aghjanian, G.K. (1979), *Eur. J. Pharmac.*, **53**, 319–328.

Guyenet, P.G., Mroz, E.A., Aghajanian, G.K. and Leeman, S.A. (1979), *Neuropharmac.*, **18**, 553–558.

Haefely, W. and Hürlimann, A. (1962), *Experientia*, **18**, 297–303.

Hanley, M.R., Lee, C.M., Jones, L.M. and Michell, R.H. (1980), *Mol. Pharmac.*, in press.

Henry, J.L. (1976), *Brain Res.*, **114**, 439–451.

Henry, J.L. (1978), *Characteristics and Function of Opioids*. (Van Ree, J.M. and Terenius, L., eds), Elsevier/North-Holland, Amsterdam, pp. 103–104.

Henry, J.L. and Ben-Ari, Y. (1976), *Brain Res.*, **117**, 540–544.

Henry, J.L., Krnjevic, K. and Morris, M.E. (1975), *Can. J. Physiol. Pharmac.*, **53**, 423–432.

Hoss, W. and Smiley, C. (1977), *J. Neurosci. Res.*, **3**, 249–256.

Iversen, L.L. (1977), *J. Neurochem.*, **29**, 5–12.

Iversen, S.D., Joyce, E.M., Kelley, A.E. and Stinus, L. (1978), *Adv. Pharmac. Ther.*, **5**, 263–272.

James, T.A. and Starr, M.S. (1977), *J. Pharm. Pharmac.*, **29**, 181–182.

James, T.A. and Starr, M.S. (1979), *Br. J. Pharmac.*, **65**, 423–429.

Johnson, A.R. and Erdös, E. (1973), *Proc. Soc. exp. biol. Med.*, **142**, 1252–1256.

Jones, L.M. and Michell, R.H. (1978), *Biochem. Soc. Trans.*, **6**, 1035–1037.

Juan, H. and Lembeck, F. (1974), *N.S. Arch. Pharmac.*, **283**, 151–164.

Katayama, Y. and North, R.A. (1978), *Nature*, **274**, 387–388.

Katz, R.J. (1979), *Neurosci. Lett.*, **12**, 133–136.

Kelley, A.E. and Iversen, S.D. (1978), *Brain Res.*, **158**, 474–478.

Kelley, A.E., Stinus, L. and Iversen, S.D. (1979), *Neurosci. Lett.*, **11**, 335–339.

Kitagawa, K., Ban, Y., Akita, T., Segawa, T., Nakata, Y. and Yajima, H. (1978), *Chem. Pharm. Bull.*, **26**, 1604–1607.

Konishi, S. and Otsuka, M. (1974a), *Nature*, **252**, 734–735.

Konishi, S. and Otsuka, M. (1974b), *Brain Res.*, **65**, 397–410.

Krivoy, W.A., Kroeger, D. and Zimmerman, E. (1977), *Substance P*. (von Euler, U.S. and Pernow, B., eds), Raven Press, New York, pp. 187–193.

Krnjevic, K. (1977), *Substance P*. (von Euler, U.S. and Pernow, B., eds), Raven Press, New York, pp. 217–230.

Krnjevic, K. and Lekic, D. (1977), *Can. J. Physiol. Pharmac.*, **55**, 958–961.

Krnjevic, K. and Morris, M.E. (1974), *Can. J. Physiol. Pharmac.*, **52**, 736–744.

Langer, S.Z. (1977), *Brit. J. Pharmac.*, **60**, 481–497.

Leeman, S.E. and Hammerschlag, R. (1967), *Endocrinol.*, **81**, 803–810.

Leeman, S. and Mroz, E. A. (1974), *Life Sci.*, **15**, 2033–2044.

Leeman, S., Mroz, E.A. and Carraway, R.E. (1977), *Peptides in Neurobiology*. (Gainer, H., ed), Plenum Press, New York, pp. 99–144.

Le Gal La Salle, G. and Ben-Ari, Y. (1977), *Brain Res.*, **135**, 174–179.

Lembeck, F. (1957), *N.S. Arch. exp. Path. Pharmak.*, **230**, 1–9.

Lembeck, F. and Gamse, R. (1977), *N.S. Arch. Pharmac.*, **299**, 295–303.

Lembeck, F. and Starke, K. (1968), *N.S. Arch. Pharmak, exp. Path.*, **259**–385.

Lembeck, F. and Zetler, G. (1962), *Int. Rev. Neurobiol.*, **4**, 159–215.

Lembeck, F., Holzer, P., Schweditsch, M. and Gamse, R. (1978a), *N.S. Arch. Pharmac.*, **305**, 9–16.

Lembeck, F., Mayer, N. and Schindler, G. (1978b), *N.S. Arch. Pharmac.*, **303**, 79–86.

Libonati, M. and Segre, G. (1960), *N.S. Arch. Pharmac.*, **240**, R14–R15.

Livett, B.G., Kozousek, V., Mizobe, F. and Dean, D.M. (1979), *Nature*, **278**, 256–257.

Loh, H.H., Cho, T.M., Wu, Y.C. and Way, E.L. (1974), *Life Sci.*, **14**, 2231–2245.

Lübke, K., Zöllner, G. and Schröder, E. (1966), *Hypotensive Peptides*. (Erdös, E., Back, N., Sicuteri, F. and Wilde A., eds), Springer-Verlag, New York, pp. 45–54.

Magnusson, T., Carlsson, A., Fisher, G.H., Chang, D. and Folkers, K. (1976), *J. neur. Trans.*, **38**, 89–93.

Malick, J.B. and Goldstein, J.M. (1978), *Life Sci.*, **23**, 835–844.

Marier, S.H., Putney, J.W. Jr., and van de Walle, C.M. (1978), *J. Physiol.*, **279**, 141–151.

Mayer, N., Lembeck, F., Saria, A. and Gamse, R. (1979), *N.S. Arch. Pharmac.*, **306**, 45–51.

Mayer, N. and Saria, A. (1979), *N.S. Arch. Pharmac.*, **307**, Supplement, R68.

Michelot, R., Leviel, V., Giorguieff-Chesselet, M.F., Chéramy, A. and Glowinski, S. (1979), *Life Sci.*, **24**, 715–724.

Michell, R. (1975), *Biochim. Biophys. Acta.* **415**, 81–147.

Mills, I.H., Macfarlane, N.A.A. and Ward, P.E. (1974), *Nature*, **247**, 108–109.

Nakata, Y., Kusaka, Y., Segawa, T., Yajima, H. and Kitagawa, K. (1978), *Life Sci.*, **22**, 259–268.

Narumi, S. and Fujita, T. (1978), *Neuropharmac.*, **17**, 73–76.

Nemeth, E.F. and Cooper, J.R. (1979), *Brain Res.*, **165**, 166–170.

Nicoll, R. (1976), *Soc. Neurosci. Symp.*, **1**, 99–122.

Nicoll, R. (1978), *J. Pharm. exp. Ther.*, **207**, 817–824.

Niedrich, H., Berseck, C. and Oehme, P. (1971), *Peptides 1969*. (Scoffone, E., ed), North-Holland, Amsterdam, pp. 370–374.

Oehme, P., Bergmann, J., Bienert, M., Hilse, H., Piesche, L., Minh Thu, P. and Scheer, E. (1977), *Substance P.* (von Euler, U.S. and Pernow, B., eds), Raven Press, New York, pp. 327–335.

Oehme, P., Bergmann, J., Müller, H., Grupe, R., Niedrich, H., Vogt, W. and Jung, F. (1972), *Acta biol. Med. Germ.*, **28**, 121–131.

Oehme, P., Bergman, J., Niedrich, H., Jung, F. and Menzel, C. (1970), *Acta biol. Med. Germ.*, **25**, 613–625.

Olpe, H.R. and Koella, W.P. (1977), *Brain Res.*, **126**, 576–579.

Otsuka, M. and Konishi, S. (1976), *Cold Spring Harbor Symp., Quant. Biol.*, **40**, 135–143.

Otsuka, M., Konishi, S., Takahashi, T. (1972a), *Proc. Jap. Acad.*, **48**, 342–346.

Otsuka, M., Konishi, S. and Takahashi, T. (1972b), *Proc. Jap. Acad.*, **48**, 747–752.

Otsuka, M., Konishi, S. and Takahashi, T. (1975), *Fed. Proc.*, **34**, 1922–1928.

Paton, W.D.M. and Zar, A.M. (1966), *Abstr. III Int. Pharmacol.* Congr. Sao Paulo, Brazil, p. 9.

Phillis, J.W. (1977), *Soc. Neurosci. Symp.*, **2**, 241–264.

Phillis, S.W. and Limacher, J.J. (1974), *Brain Res.*, **69**, 158–163.

Puil, E., Krnjevic, K. and Werman, R. (1976), *Fed. Proc.* **35**, 307.

Putney, J.W. Jr., (1979), *Pharmac. Rev.*, **30**, 209–245.

Quik, M., Iversen, L.L. and Bloom, S.R. (1978), *Biochem. Pharmac.*, **27**, 2209–2213.

Randic, M. and Miletic, V. (1977), *Brain Res.*, **128**, 164–169.

Reubi, J.-C., Emson, P.C., Jessell, T.M. and Iversen, L.L. (1978), *N.S. Arch. Pharmac.*, **304**, 271–275.

Rietschoten, J. van, Tregear, G., Leeman, S., Powell, D., Niall, H. and Potts, J.T. (1975), *Peptides 1974*. (Wolman, Y. and Wiley, J., eds), North-Holland, Amsterdam, pp. 113–115.

Roberts, M.H.T. and Wright, D.M. (1978), *J. Physiol.*, **281**, 33–34P.

Rondeau, D.B., Jolicoeur, F.B., Belanger, F. and Barbeau, A. (1978), *Pharmac, Biochem. Behav.*, **9**, 769–775.

Rosell, S., Bjökroth, U., Change, D., Yamaguchi, I., Wan, Y.P., Rackur, G., Fisher, G. and Folkers, K. (1977), *Substance P*. (von Euler, U.S. and Pernow, B., eds), Raven Press, New York, pp. 83–88.

Rudich, L. and Butcher, F.R. (1976), *Biochim. Biophys. Acta.*, **444**, 704–711.

Ryall, R.W. and Belcher, G. (1977), *Brain Res.*, **137**, 376–380.

Saito, K., Konishi, S. and Otsuka, M. (1975a), *Jap. J. Pharmac.*, **25**, 73P–74P.

Saito, K., Konishi, S. and Otsuka, M. (1975b), *Brain Res.*, **97**, 177–180.

Sandberg, B. and Lee, C.M. (1979), *Regulation and Function of Neural Peptides*. Brescia, Italy.

Sandrin, E. and Boissonnas, R. (1964), *Helv. Chim. Acta.*, **47**, 1294–1332.

Saria, A., Mayer, N., Gamse, R. and Lembeck, F. (1978), *Proc. Eur. Soc. Neurochem.*, **1**, 464.

Sastry, B.R. (1978), *Brain Res.*, **144**, 404–410.

Schröder, E., Lübke, K. and Hempel, R. (1965), *Experientia*, **21**, 70–71.

Segawa, T., Nakata, Y., Nakamura, K., Yajima, H. and Kitagawa, K. (1976), *Jap. J. Pharmac.*, **26**, 757–760.

Segawa, T., Nakata, Y., Yajima, H. and Kitagawa, K. (1977), *Jap. J. Pharmac.*, **27**, 573–580.

Sheppard, M.C., Kronheim, S. and Pimstone, B.L. (1979), *J. Neurochem.*, **32**, 647–649.

Silbergeld, E.K. and Walters, J.R. (1979), *Neurosci. Lett.*, **12**, 119–126.

Skrabanek, P. and Powell, D. (1978), *Substance P*, Vol. 1. Churchill Livinstone, Edinburgh.

Spearman, T.N. and Pritchard, E.T. (1977), *Biochim. Biophys. Acta.*, **466**, 198–207.

Starr, M.S. (1978), *K. Pharm. Pharmac.*, **30**, 359–363.

Starr, M.S., James, T.A. and Gaytten, D. (1978), *Eur. J. Pharmac.*, **48**, 203–212.

Steinacker, A. (1977), *Nature*, **267**, 268–270.

Steinacker, A. and Highstein, S.M. (1976), *Brain Res.*, **114**, 128–133.

Stern, P. and Dobric, V. (1957), *Psychotropic Drugs*, (Garattini, S. and Ghetti, V., eds), Elsevier, Amsterdam, pp. 448–452.

Stern, P. and Hadzovic, J. (1973), *Arch. Int. Pharmacodyn.*, **202**, 259–262.

Stern, P. and Hukovic, S. (1960), *Med. Exp.*, **2**, 1–7.

Stern, P., Catovic, S. and Stern, M. (1974), *N.S. Arch. Pharmac.*, **281**, 233–239.

Stewart, J.M., Getto, C.J., Neldner, K., Reeve, E.B., Krivoy, W.A. and Zimmermann, E. (1976), *Nature*, **262**, 784–785.

Stinus, L., Kelley, A.E. and Iversen, S.D. (1978), *Nature*, **276**, 616–618.

Studer, R.O., Trzeciak, A. and Lergier, W. (1973), *Helv. Chim. Acta.*, **56**, 860–866.

Terenius, L. (1976), *J. Pharm. Pharmac.*, **27**, 450–452.

Traczyk, W. (1977), *Substance P.* (von Euler, U.S. and Pernow, B., eds), Raven Press, New York, pp. 297–309.

Vincent, J.-D. and Barker, J.L. (1979), *Science*, **205**, 1409–1412.

Walaszek, E.J. and Dyer, D.C. (1966), *Hypotensive Peptides*, (Erdös, E.G., Back, N. Sicuteri, F. and Wilde, A.F., eds), Springer-Verlag, Berlin, pp. 329–340.

Waldmeier, P.C., Kam, R. and Stöcklin, K. (1978), *Brain Res.*, **159**, 223–227.

Walker, A.J., Kemp, J.A., Yajima, H., Kitagawa, K. and Woodruff, G.N. (1976), *Experientia*, **32**, 214–215.

Wheeler, C.S., Van de Walle, C.M. and Putney, J.W. (1979), *Fed. Proc.*, **38**, 1039.

Wilson, P.R. and Yaksh, T.L. (1978), *Eur. J. Pharmac.*, **51**, 323–330.

Wright, D.M. and Roberts, M.H.T. (1978), *Life Sci.*, **22**, 19–24.

Yajima, H., Kitagawa, K. and Segawa, T. (1973), *Chem. Pharm. Bull.*, **21**, 682–683.

Yamaguchi, I., Rackur, G., Leban, J.J., Björkroth, U., Rosell, S. and Folkers, K. (1979), *Acta. Chem. Scand.*, **33**, 63–68.

Yanaihara, N., Yanaihara, C., Horihashi, M., Sato, H., Iizuka, Y., Hashimoto, T. and Sakagami, M. (1977), *Substance P.* (von Euler, U.S. and Pernow, B., eds), Raven Press, New York, pp. 27–33.

Zetler, G. (1956), *N.S. Arch. Pharmac.*, **228**, 513–538.

Zieglgänsberger, W. and Tulloch, I.F. (1979), *Brain Res.*, **166**, 273–282.

Note added in proof

Since completing this review, we have prepared (^{3}H)–SP of high specific activity and find that it binds with high affinity (K_d = 0.4 nM) to saturable sites (B_{max} = 27 fmol/mg protein) in rat brain membrane preparations. The structural specificity of these sites is restricted to biologically active analogues of SP, suggesting that they represent SP receptors in CNS (M.R. Hanley, B.E. Sandberg, C.M. Lee, L.L. Iversen, D.E. Brundish and R. Wade, *Nature* – in press).

4 Enkephalin and Endorphin Receptors

STEVEN R. CHILDERS

Acknowledgements
I thank Solomon H. Snyder for valuable suggestions and encouragement,
and Pamela Morgan for preparation of the manuscript.

Neurotransmitter Receptors Part 1
(*Receptors and Recognition*, Series B, Volume 9)
Edited by S.J. Enna and H.I. Yamamura
Published in 1980 by Chapman and Hall, 11 New Fetter Lane,
London EC4P 4EE
© Chapman and Hall

4.1 INTRODUCTION

The actions of a variety of CNS-active drugs are mediated through interactions at the level of specific neurotransmitter receptors. This is certainly true for the opiate narcotics, which exert their principal effects by interacting with receptors whose endogenous ligands are opioid peptides such as enkephalin and β-endorphin. This conclusion has been obtained by two general advances of research. The first, in 1973, was the finding that labeled opiate drugs bound stereospecifically and with high affinity to receptor sites in brain membranes. The second advance occurred in 1975 with the discovery that opiate-like substances existed in brain and were characterized as peptides, including the pentapeptide enkephalins and later, the 31-amino acid peptide β-endorphin. The properties of this new class of neurotransmitter candidates have been described by a vast explosion of literature of which this review can cover a small portion. The emphasis of this review will be on the interactions of these peptides with receptor binding sites and on recent information exploring whether the peptides display the properties of typical neurotransmitters. A number of recent reviews cover the details of other aspects of opiate receptors and opioid peptides (Fredrickson, 1977; Miller and Cuatrecascas, 1978; Simon and Hiller, 1978; Terenius, 1978; Uhl *et al.*, 1978a; Snyder and Childers, 1979).

4.2 OPIATE PHARMACOLOGY AND THE RECEPTOR CONCEPT

The existence of opiate receptor binding sites in brain was suspected many years before their actual identification because of the well-known pharmacological properties of the opiate alkaloids. Morphine was first isolated from opium in 1803 and its structural formula was correctly proposed in 1925. Since then morphine has been subjected to an endless series of chemical transformations in attempts to synthesize the 'perfect analgesic', free of the adverse side effects of dependence, tolerance, and respiratory depression which characterize the parent compound. Although the 'perfect analgesic' is yet to be found, the numerous structure–activity studies which resulted from the search have provided invaluable insight that opiate effects are mediated by interactions with specific receptors. First, although morphine itself is not a highly potent analgesic (usual human dose is 2 to 15 mg i.v.), many of its derivatives are extremely potent. One example is etorphine, whose effective analgesic dose of 120 to 200 µg (i.v.)

places it in a class with LSD as one of the most potent psycho-active drugs known. Such an activity suggests that the drug is combining with high affinity to specific receptor sites. Other modifications of the opiate chemical structure can transform an agonist into an antagonist. Many such changes involve relatively small structural alterations: e.g. substitution of the *N*-methyl group of the potent agonist oxymorphone by an *N*-allyl group results in the formation of the pure antagonist naloxone, which produces no analgesic activity on its own but effectively blocks the actions of opiate agonists. The existence of antagonists supports the concept of specific receptors which would bind both classes of drug, although only the agonist class would bind in such a way as to elicit a physiological response. Other chemical modifications of opiates produce the mixed agonist–antagonists which, depending on the dose, display characteristics of each class. Some of these drugs can be less addicting than pure agonists and have therefore been useful clinically. Finally, the actions of many opiates are stereospecific, with the levo or (−)-isomer being thousands of times more potent than the dextro (+)-isomer.

The early efforts to identify specific opiate receptors by biochemical techniques utilized these specific pharmacological properties to screen the binding of radioactive drugs to brain membranes. Goldstein *et al.* (1971) described binding of ^{3}H-levorphanol to mouse brain homogenates, of which only 2 per cent was displaced by active stereoisomers. The low specific binding in these early experiments was the result of the low specific radioactivity of the labelled ligands which were available at the time. In fact, further purification of such binding revealed that the sites involved cerebroside sulfate and not the pharmacologically relevant opiate receptor (Loh *et al.*, 1974). The development of labeled drugs with higher specific radioactivity led to the demonstration of specific, high-affinity binding of ^{3}H-opiates to mammalian brain membranes using ^{3}H-naloxone (Pert and Snyder, 1973a; Terenius, 1973) and ^{3}H-etorphine (Simon *et al.*, 1973). Specific *in vitro* binding of labeled drugs to receptors could only be observed if several technical requirements were fulfilled, including the use of low concentrations of ligand to maximize high-affinity binding and the rapid separation of bound and free ligand binding. The latter requirement has been fulfilled by either rapid filtration through glass fiber filters or by centrifugation. A complete review of the technical requirements for receptor binding has been compiled by Bennett (1978).

Further studies using these techniques have confirmed that *in vitro* binding experiments identify physiologically relevant opiate receptor sites. These basic characteristics are summarized below.

(1) Binding of labeled opiates is saturable at low concentrations of ligand, with equilibrium dissociation constants of most opiates calculated at 1 nM or less (Pert and Snyder, 1973b; Snyder *et al.*, 1975). The use of ^{3}H-opiates

with specific radioactivity of at least 20 Ci/mmol in equilibrium binding experiments usually reveals the existence of both high- and low-affinity binding sites (Pasternak and Snyder, 1975b). For example, Scatchard analysis of ^{3}H-naloxone binding calculates high-affinity K_d of 0.4 nM and low-affinity K_d of 5 nM.

(2) Binding of opiates is stereospecific, paralleling the pharmacological activities of these drugs. For example, the analgesic levorphanol is 4000 times more potent than its inactive stereoisomer dextrorphan in displacing ^{3}H-naloxone binding (Pert and Snyder, 1973a).

(3) In general, opiate receptor binding is pharmacologically relevant, since the relative potencies of many opiates in displacing ^{3}H-opiate binding can be correlated with their pharmacological potencies (Pert and Snyder, 1973b; Snyder *et al.*, 1975). Etorphine, one of the most potent opiate analgesics, has 20 times the affinity of morphine in displacing ^{3}H-naloxone. Propoxyphene, a very weak analgesic, has only 1/200 of the affinity of morphine in binding studies. However, a detailed examination shows that good correlation between analgesia and binding studies does not exist because each drug has its own *in vivo* metabolic and pharmacokinetic properties which cannot be measured by *in vitro* experiments. One case is etorphine, which is 100 to 10 000 times more potent than morphine *in vivo*, yet is only 20 times more potent in receptor binding. A large part of the pharmacological potency of etorphine is undoubtably due to its extreme lipophilic structure which enables it to cross the blood–brain barrier with relative ease. Such examples point out the difficulty in comparing data from biochemical assays with those from behavioral tests of analgesia. Nevertheless, opiate receptor binding studies can be closely correlated with pharmacological potencies of opiates in another tissue, the guinea-pig ileum. Studies by Paton (1957) and others (Kosterlitz and Waterfield, 1975) have shown that opiate agonists inhibit the electrically induced contractions of the guinea-pig ileum, and that opiate antagonists specifically reverse this effect. Since the ileum also contains ^{3}H-opiate binding sites (Pert and Snyder, 1973b), Creese and Snyder (1975) were able to observe a close correlation between the affinity of drugs in displacing ^{3}H-naloxone binding and in their pharmacological potencies in strips of the guinea-pig ileum.

(4) The distribution of opiate receptor binding is highly specific. Specific binding is highest in brain and not apparent in many non-nervous tissues (Pert and Snyder, 1973a). This is best seen in the ileum, where binding is abolished upon removal of the nerve plexus (Pert and Snyder, 1973b).

These basic series of experiments, conducted mainly between 1973 and 1975, clearly established the relevancy of *in vitro* opiate receptor binding studies and suggested that many, if not all, opiate physiological effects are mediated by receptor interactions.

4.3 ENDOGENOUS OPIOID PEPTIDES

4.3.1 Nomenclature

The development of a new research area inevitably leads to a confusing variety of terms.

Most researchers have agreed upon the naming of two groups of opioid peptides: enkephalins and pituitary endorphins. The term enkephalin refers to two pentapeptides, methionine-enkephalin (met-enkephalin), H_2N-tyr-gly-gly-phe-met-OH, and leucine–enkephalin (leu-enkephalin) H_2N-tyr-gly-gly-phe-leu-OH. The amino acid sequence of met-enkephalin is contained within the sequence of the 91-amino acid polypeptide β-lipotropin (β-LPH) isolated from pituitary and represents amino acids 61–65. The 31-amino acid C-terminal fragment of β-LPH (amino acids 61–91) is a potent opioid peptide generally known as β-endorphin or C-fragment. Other fragments of β-LPH that possess opioid activity include α-endorphin (β-LPH$_{61-76}$), γ-endorphin (β-LPH$_{61-77}$) and C'-fragment (β-LPH$_{61-87}$). The amino acid sequences of these peptides are represented in Fig. 4.1.

4.3.2 Identification and isolation

The discovery of opioid peptides was not accidental since their existence was suggested by the discovery of opiate receptors themselves. It did not seem reasonable that animals would develop receptors to opiates, compounds which most animals never see, unless they already possessed an endogenous opioid system that interacted with opiate receptors in the absence of drugs. Direct evidence for the concept of endogenous opioids came from the discovery (Reynolds, 1969; Mayer and Liebeskind, 1974) that electrical stimulation of the central gray in the brainstem produces analgesia. Moreover, in rats the stimulation analgesia can be reversed by naloxone (Akil *et al.*, 1976) suggesting that stimulation could be releasing endogenous analgesic substances in the brain whose effects at the opiate receptor are blocked by opiate antagonists. Finally, *in vitro* experiments showed that opiate receptor binding was increased by prior injection of either agonists or

Leu-enkephalin	H-Tyr-Gly-Gly-Phe-Leu-OH
Met-enkephalin	H-Tyr-Gly-Gly-Phe-Met-OH
α-endorphin	H-Tyr-Gly-Gly-Phe-Met-Thr-Ser-Glu-Lys-Ser-Gln-Thr-Pro-Leu-Val-Thr-OH
γ-endorphin	H-Tyr-Gly-Gly-Phe-Met-Thr-Ser-Glu-Lys-Ser-Gln-Thr-Pro-Leu-Val-Thr-Leu-O┐
β-endorphin	H-Tyr-Gly-Gly-Phe-Met-Thr-Ser-Glu-Lys-Ser-Gln-Thr-Pro-Leu-Val-Thr-Leu-Ph
	Lys-Asn-Ala-Ile-Ile-Lys-Asn-Ala-Tyr-Lys-Lys-Gly-Glu-OH

Fig. 4.1 Amino acid sequences of opioid peptides, including human β-endorphin. Underlined portion represents residues 61–65 of β-LPH.

antagonists (Pert and Snyder, 1976) or by incubation of brain extracts at 37° C (Pasternak *et al.*, 1975b), indicating a displacement of endogenously bound ligands.

Two methods were used to isolate the presumed opioid substances. Hughes (1975) screened for the ability of brain extracts to mimic the influence of morphine upon electrically induced contractions of the mouse vas deferens and the guinea-pig ileum. Moreover, Pasternak *et al.* (1975c) and Terenius and Wahlstrom (1974) demonstrated that brain extracts contained a substance that competed for opiate receptor binding. Specificity of these methods was established by showing that the marked regional variations in opiate receptors in brain were paralleled by similar variations in the concentration of the morphine-like substance (Hughes, 1975; Pasternak *et al.*, 1976).

With these methods it was possible to differentiate artefacts from the true opioid substances and to purify them. Hughes *et al.* (1975) purified the substance from pig brain and found it to consist of a mixture of two pentapeptides, met-enkephalin and leu-enkephalin. These structures were confirmed by Simantov and Snyder (1976a) using calf brain as a source of the peptides and displacement of ^{3}H-naloxone binding as an assay. The amino acid sequence of met-enkephalin was soon found (Hughes *et al.*, 1975) within the sequence of the 91-amino acid pituitary polypeptide β-lipotropin (β-LPH) originally isolated by Li (1964). Already, opioid peptides larger than enkephalin were being discovered in pituitary extracts (Cox *et al.*, 1975), so a major question was whether other fragments of β-LPH may also possess opioid activity. Several groups reported that the C-terminal 31 amino acids of β-LPH, named β-endorphin, was a potent opioid peptide in both receptor binding assays and in bioassays using guinea-pig ileum and mouse vas deferens (Bradbury *et al.*, 1976a, b, c; Chretien *et al.*, 1976; Cox *et al.*, 1976; Li and Chung, 1976). Other fragments of β-LPH also possess some opioid activity (e.g. α-, γ-endorphin) and all such peptides, including β-endorphin, incorporate the sequence of met-enkephalin. The parent molecule, β-LPH, has no significant opioid activity.

Other workers (Gintzler *et al.*, 1976) have detected a non-peptide opioid substance in brain which cross-reacts with morphine antisera. Although its chemical identity is not yet known, this morphine-like compound (MLC) presumably has a structure related to morphine. MLC is potent in displacing ^{3}H-leu-enkephalin binding to neuroblastoma X glioma cells (Blume *et al.*, 1977), although its exact potency is unknown because of its incomplete chemical characterization. The regional distribution of MLC, measured by immunocytochemistry, is different from that of enkephalin, β-endorphin and opiate receptors (Gintzler *et al.*, 1978); in particular, MLC-reactive cells are found in the cerebellum, an area which contains no appreciable enkephalin and very little opiate receptor binding.

4.3.3 Assay procedures

The original techniques used to assay opioid peptides took advantage of their opiate-like properties either in inhibiting electrically induced contractions of the guinea-pig ileum and mouse vas deferens (Hughes, 1975), or in competing with ^{3}H-opiates in receptor binding studies (Pasternak *et al.*, 1975c). The potencies of the peptides in these assay systems are compared with morphine in Table 4.1. One disadvantage of the opiate assays for the peptides is the possibility that nonspecific factors can interfere with the binding assay. For example, Simantov *et al.* (1977) found nonspecific receptor-active substances distributed evenly throughout rat brain. A second disadvantage is that the opiate assays cannot discriminate the various opioid peptides from each other or from administered opiate drugs. This disadvantage can be circumvented by procedures which chemically separate various components, followed by standard opiate assays. High-pressure liquid chromatography has been effective in separating met- and leu-enkephalin from each other as well as from other fragments of β-LPH (Rubinstein *et al.*, 1977; Meek and Bohan, 1978; Loeber *et al.*, 1979). For addiction experiments, Childers *et al.* (1977) developed an ion-exchange method to separate morphine and naloxone from opioid peptides. Finally, Smith *et al.* (1976) utilized cyanogen bromide to selectively destroy met-enkephalin without affecting leu-enkephalin.

Another approach to differentiate enkephalins and endorphins is to

Table 4.1 Potencies of opioid peptides in different opiate assays.

Substance	Relative potency (morphine = 1)			
	Guinea-pig ileum	Mouse vas deferens	^{3}H-naloxone (brain)	Analgesia (i.c.v.)
Morphine	1.0	1.0	1.0	1.0
Natural opioid peptides				
met-enkephalin	0.72	42	0.60	0.015
leu-enkephalin	0.15	67	0.51	0.005
α-endorphin	0.32	17	0.075	>0.10
β-endorphin	0.88	8.3	2.0	33
Synthetic peptides				
D-ala$_2$-met-enkephalin	4.3	230	0.52	3
FK-33-824			1.5	1000

Relative potency ratios were calculated from the data of Lord *et al.* (1977), Childers *et al.* (1979), Roemer *et al.* (1977), Loh *et al.* (1976) and Belluzzi *et al.* (1976). Other studies may provide slightly different results.

prepare specific radioimmunoassays. Enkephalin radioimmunoassays have been prepared by many groups (Simantov and Snyder, 1976b; Weissman *et al.*, 1976; Yang *et al.*, 1977; Miller *et al.*, 1978a); these assays effectively differentiate met-enkephalin from leu-enkephalin, as well as enkephalin from β-endorphin.

More recently, radioimmunoassays for β-endorphin have also been developed (Guillemin *et al.*, 1977a; LaBella *et al.*, 1977; Li *et al.*, 1977; Snell *et al.*, 1977; Watson *et al.*, 1977). Although these antisera readily distinguish β-endorphin from the enkephalins, they display considerable cross-reactivity with β-LPH. After separation of β-endorphin and β-LPH by gel filtration, radioimmunoassays have shown that levels of β-endorphin in brain are considerably lower than those of enkephalins, while β-endorphin predominates in pituitary (Rossier *et al.*, 1977b).

4.4 PROPERTIES OF OPIATE RECEPTORS

The discovery of the endogenous opioid peptides indicated that the 'opiate receptors' can perhaps more accurately be termed enkephalin and endorphin receptors. With this in mind, this section will discuss the details of the binding of opiates compared to enkephalin and endorphins, including factors which regulate binding, structure–activity relationships, and the concept of multiple opiate receptors.

4.4.1 Enkephalin binding and stable enkephalin analogs

As shown in Table 4.1, both met- and leu-enkephalin are potent in binding to various receptor preparations. In the case of the ileum and vas deferens bioassays, the specificity of enkephalin interaction is further demonstrated by the complete reversal of their inhibition of contractions by naloxone (Smith *et al.*, 1976). In brain, unlabeled enkephalins displace ³H-naloxone binding with typical non-co-operative displacement curves with Hill coefficients approximating 1 (Simantov and Snyder, 1976a, c).

One problem in measuring enkephalin by radioreceptor assay is the rapid degradation of enkephalin that occurs at 25 and 37° C in the presence of brain membranes. Degradation of enkephalin can be prevented by the addition of the antibiotics bacitractin (Simantov and Snyder, 1976c; Miller *et al.*, 1977) or puromycin (Knight and Klee, 1978). Alternatively, incubations can be carried out at 0° C (Simantov and Snyder, 1976c). Further studies of enkephalin degradation (Hambrook *et al.*, 1976) showed that rapid destruction occurs in human plasma as well as rat brain. Examination of degradation products by thin layer chromatography showed that deactivation occurs with cleavage of the tyr-gly amide bond by

aminopeptidase activity. Attempts were made by Pert *et al.* (1976a) to
stabilize this bond by the substitution of gly_2 by a D-amino acid that would
presumably block the accessibility of this crucial bond to proteolytic
enzymes. The introduction of D-ala into position 2, thus creating
D-ala_2-met-enkephalin, produces an analog with an equivalent potency to
met-enkephalin in receptor binding, but which is not degraded. Other
enkephalin analogs also resist proteolytic degradation: FK-33-824
(H_2N-tyr-D-ala-gly-(CH_3)-phe-met(o)-ol) (see Table 4.1) (Roemer *et al.*,
1977), and H_2N-tyr-D-met-gly-phe-pro-NH_2 (Bajusz *et al.*, 1977). Marks *et
al.* (1978) have synthesized a pentafluoro phenylalanine derivative of D-ala
enkephalin which is also extremely resistant to proteolysis presumably
because the *C*-terminal end of the peptide is also protected. β-endorphin,
unlike enkephalin, is relatively stable in the presence of both plasma and
brain membranes, which explains its high analgesic potency (Graf *et al.*,
1976). Nevertheless, β-endorphin can be degraded by brain homogenates
and this breakdown can also be inhibited by bacitracin (Patthy *et al.*, 1977).
The possible physiological role of the hydrolysis of opioid peptides will be
discussed later.

More details about enkephalin binding have been obtained with the use of
^{3}H-enkephalin as a ligand (Simantov and Snyder, 1976b; Morin *et al.*, 1976;
Audigier *et al.*, 1977; Lord *et al.*, 1977; Simantov *et al.*, 1978).
^{3}H-Met-enkephalin binding to rat brain membranes is saturable, with half
maximal binding at a concentration of 1 nM. Scatchard analysis reveals two
distinct linear components with a higher affinity dissociation constant of
0.64 nM and lower affinity dissociation constant of 2.6 nM. Binding of
^{3}H-met-enkephalin is also stereospecific, with levorphanol 10 000-fold more
potent in displacing ^{3}H-met-enkephalin than dextrorphan (Simantov *et al.*,
1978).

Miller *et al.* (1978b) have prepared ^{125}I-D-ala-enkephalin and showed that
the mono-iodo derivative possesses high-affinity binding ($K_D = 0.8$ nM).
Since ^{125}I-labeled compounds have far greater specific activity than
^{3}H-labeled derivatives, they can be utilized in more sensitive receptor assays.

Until recently, studies with labeled β-endorphin in binding experiments
have been impossible because ^{125}I-β-endorphin has no binding activity in
receptor studies. However, Houghten and Li (1978) have synthesized
^{3}H-β-endorphin which binds to guinea-pig ileum with an IC_{50} of 7 nM. In
addition, ^{125}I-D-ala_2-β-endorphin has recently been prepared by methods
such that significant binding could be detected in brain (Hazum *et al.*, 1979).

4.4.2 Regulation of agonist and antagonist binding by ions and nucleotides

An early goal of receptor binding studies was to determine whether opiate
receptors could distinguish between agonist and antagonist binding. In

Table 4.2 Agents which differentiate opiate agonist and antagonist binding.

| Agent | Effects on: | |
	^{3}H-agonist binding	^{3}H-antagonist binding
Monovalent cations		
Na$^+$, Li$^+$	↓↓	↑
K$^+$, Cs$^+$	None	None
Divalent cations		
Mn^{2+}	↑	None
Mg^{2+}, Ca^{2+} (higher conc.)	↑	None
Enzymes		
Trypsin	↓↓	↓
Phospholipase A	↓↓	↓
Phospholipases C, D	None	None
Neuramididase	None	None
Sulfhydryl reagents	↓↓	↓
Nucleotides		
GTP, GDP	↓↓	None
GMP, ATP, etc.	None	None

normal, untreated membranes, in the absence of ions and nucleotides, no differences can be detected in the relative affinities of agonists and antagonists. However, a number of treatments can alter binding to effectively differentiate agonists and antagonists. These treatments are summarized in Table 4.2.

One of the most dramatic differences in agonist and antagonist binding occurs in the presence of sodium. At relatively low concentrations (as little as 0.5 mM), sodium causes a decrease in ^{3}H-agonist binding and a slight increase in ^{3}H-antagonist binding (Pert *et al.*, 1978; Pert and Snyder, 1974; Simon *et al.*, 1975b). The effect is specific for sodium, since only lithium (whose atomic radius is close to that of sodium) and not potassium, cesium and rubidium, mimics the effect of sodium on agonist and antagonist binding. The effectiveness of sodium was demonstrated by studies which measured the potencies of unlabeled drugs in inhibiting ^{3}H-naloxone binding in the presence and absence of sodium (Pert *et al.*, 1973; Pert and Snyder, 1974). Pure antagonists are just as potent in the presence as in the absence of sodium, while pure agonists become 12 to 60 times weaker and mixed agonist-antagonists are moderately (3 to 6 fold) weaker in the presence of sodium. This 'sodium index' of opiates has been useful in screening large numbers of drugs for therapeutic potential as analgesics. Interestingly, both met- and leu-enkephalin, as well as β-endorphin, which act as pure agonists in the guinea-pig ileum bioassay, display 6 to 10 fold reductions in potency in the presence of sodium, and therefore are affected more like mixed agonist–antagonists (Childers *et al.*, 1979). Changes in the sequence of enkephalin result in large changes in the sodium index of the peptide analogs (Beddell *et al.*, 1977), indicating that sodium alone is not effective in predicting agonist profiles of enkephalin analogs.

Detailed biochemical studies have examined the mechanism of the sodium effect on the opiate receptor. In equilibrium binding studies, sodium selectively abolishes high-affinity sites with no effect on low-affinity sites (Pasternak and Snyder, 1975b). Thus, depending on the concentration of ^{3}H-ligand used, the effect would appear as either a decrease in the number (Pert and Snyder, 1974) or affinity (Simon *et al.*, 1975b) of sites. In kinetic experiments, sodium increases the dissociation of ^{3}H-agonists with no effect on the dissociation of ^{3}H-antagonists (Pert and Snyder, 1974; Simon *et al.*, 1975b; Simantov *et al.*, 1978). The slight increase in ^{3}H-antagonist binding in the presence of sodium appears to be elicited at least in part by an accelerated dissociation of endogenous opiate peptides from receptor sites (Pasternak *et al.*, 1975b; Pasternak *et al.* 1976). This idea is supported by the finding that sodium increases dissociation of ^{3}H-enkephalin binding in the same way as other ^{3}H-agonists (Simantov *et al.*, 1978).

Divalent cations also differentiate agonist and antagonist binding (Pasternak *et al.*, 1975a; Simantov *et al.*, 1976a). Low concentrations of manganese and magnesium, but not calcium, selectively increase ^{3}H-agonist binding with no effect on ^{3}H-antagonist binding. The effects of manganese are more pronounced in the presence of sodium. These results may be of physiological significance since manganese enhances the pharmacological actions of morphine on cat nictitating membrane (Enero, 1977).

Various treatments to brain membranes can also cause differences between agonist and antagonist binding. Binding of ^{3}H-agonists is extremely sensitive to degradation by enzymes such as trypsin and phospholipase A, while ^{3}H-antagonist binding is not as severely affected (Pasternak and Snyder, 1975a). Similarly, agonist binding is more drastically inhibited by protein modifying reagents such as iodoacetamide, N-ethymaleimide and p-mercuribenzoate (Pasternak *et al.*, 1975b).

Recent studies indicate that guanine nucleotides could be physiological regulators of opiate agonist interactions. In other receptor systems (Mukherjee and Lefkowitz, 1976; Lad *et al.*, 1977; Lefkowitz and Williams, 1977) GTP plays a dual role in coupling receptors to adenylate cyclase, as well as sensitizing receptors by decreasing affinity and increasing dissociation rates of agonists. Thus, the agonist is removed and the receptor is sensitized for further interactions. In these receptor systems, GTP has no effect on the binding of antagonists. Recently, Blume (1978a, b) described GTP-induced decrease in ^{3}H-agonist binding to opiate receptors in both brain membranes and neuroblastoma X glioma hybrid cells. Although the effect of GTP was specific (not seen with GMP or any adenine nucleotides), the study showed that GTP decreased binding of antagonists as well as agonists. Nevertheless, other studies (Childers and Snyder, 1978) demonstrated that GTP could differentiate agonist and antagonist binding; i.e. in the presence of sodium, GTP decreased only ^{3}H-agonist binding. This differentiation was confirmed by examining the potencies of various opiates in displacing ^{3}H-diprenorphine binding in the presence and absence of both GTP and sodium. Under these conditions, agonists and antagonists were differentiated more dramatically than in the presence of sodium alone, and in particular the potencies of enkephalins were reduced to a greater degree than any opiate tested (Childers and Snyder, 1980).

The details of GTP–opiate interactions have also been studied (Blume, 1978a; Childers and Snyder, 1980). In equilibrium binding experiments, the actions of sodium and GTP are additive, and together they completely abolish high-affinity agonist binding sites. At lower concentrations, GTP lowers the number of binding sites without affecting affinity. In kinetic experiments, GTP increases both the association and dissociation rates of agonists. Thus, the principal action of guanine nucleotides is to increase both the on-rate and the off-rate of agonists, thereby increasing the availability of receptors as in other systems.

If GTP directly affects opiate receptor interactions with agonists, it may also serve to couple opiate receptors with adenylate cyclase. It is well known that opiate agonists inhibit prostaglandin E_1-stimulated adenylate cyclase in brain homogenates (Collier and Roy, 1974) and in neuroblastoma X glioma cells (Sharma *et al.*, 1975; Traber *et al.*, 1975); these effects are blocked by naloxone. Enkephalin also inhibits prostaglandin-stimulated adenylate cyclase and increases cyclic GMP levels in striatal slices (Minneman and Iversen, 1976) and inhibits basal adenylate cyclase in neuroblastoma X glioma cells (Klee and Nirenberg, 1976). Preliminary data (A.J. Blume, personal communication) indicate that the degree of enkephalin-inhibited adenylate cyclase in neuroblastoma X glioma depends on the presence of GTP. If these results are confirmed they suggest that at least some opiate receptors may be coupled to adenylate cyclase and, analogous to other receptors systems, the receptor-cyclase coupling may be GTP-dependent.

4.4.3 Structure–activity studies

(a) Enkephalin
The production of synthetic analogs of enkephalin has led to extensive structure–activity studies to determine which amino acid residues are

required for receptor binding. Of primary importance is an unaltered
N-terminal tyrosine; removal of the tyrosine amino or hydroxyl groups
eliminates opioid activity (Buscher *et al.*, 1976; Chang *et al.*, 1976;
Fredrickson *et al.*, 1976; Morgan *et al.*, 1976; Terenius *et al.*, 1976).
Phenylalanine in position 4 is also crucial (Morgan *et al.*, 1976); replacing
phenylalanine with tyrosine results in an almost total loss of activity. Loss
of activity is also seen if the distance between the aromatic residues is
altered (Terenius *et al.*, 1976); the gly in position 3 seems particularly
crucial (Beddell *et al.*, 1977). Alterations in the *C*-terminal portion also
reduce activity, although this portion of the molecule is less crucial than
the *N*-terminal moiety. In particular, activity depends on a hydrophobic
C-terminal residue, since increasing hydrophilicity on this residue decreases
activity (Beddell *et al.*, 1977). Therefore, from these structure–activity
studies it is apparent that the biological activity of enkephalin will not
tolerate significant substitutions with natural amino acids. However,
substitution with unnatural amino acids, in particular D-ala for gly_2,
appears to relieve some of these restrictions, especially on the tyr residue.
For example, both iodo-tyr_1-D-ala_2 enkephalin (Miller *et al.*, 1978b) and
N-methyl-tyr_1-D-ala_2 enkephalin (Roemer and Pless, 1979) are active.

Both chemical conformation and biological activity studies have been
utilized to determine the three-dimensional active structure of enkephalin.
Details of various structure models have been reviewed by Gorin *et al.*
(1978). A number of workers have devised conformations of enkephalin
based on theoretical minimum-energy calculations (Isogai *et al.*, 1977;
Loew and Burt, 1978), proton magnetic resonance experiments of
enkephalin in solution (Jones *et al.*, 1976; Roques *et al.*, 1976) and X-ray
diffraction of enkephalin in crystalline form (Smith and Griffin, 1978). A
basic problem of all such studies is the possibility that the conformation
seen in solution or in crystal form may not be relevant to the actual
conformation of enkephalin at the active site of the opiate receptor.
Indeed, the calculations of Loew and Burt (1978) indicate that the
theoretical minimum-energy conformation does not resemble the structure
of morphine, and that significant increases in energy are required for
enkephalin to adopt a tyramine conformation like morphine. Therefore, it
is important that physical measurements and theoretical calculations be
combined with structure–activity studies in order to construct an accurate
model of the structure of enkephalin. As yet there is no consensus
concerning the details of such a model, but one point is clear: the tyr
residue of enkephalin corresponds to the tyramine ring A moiety of
morphine (Fig. 4.2). This conclusion is based principally upon the data that
both the hydroxyl group (corresponding to ring A hydroxyl)
and the amino group (corresponding to the *N*-methyl group on
morphine) of tyrosine are required for activity. The absolute configuration

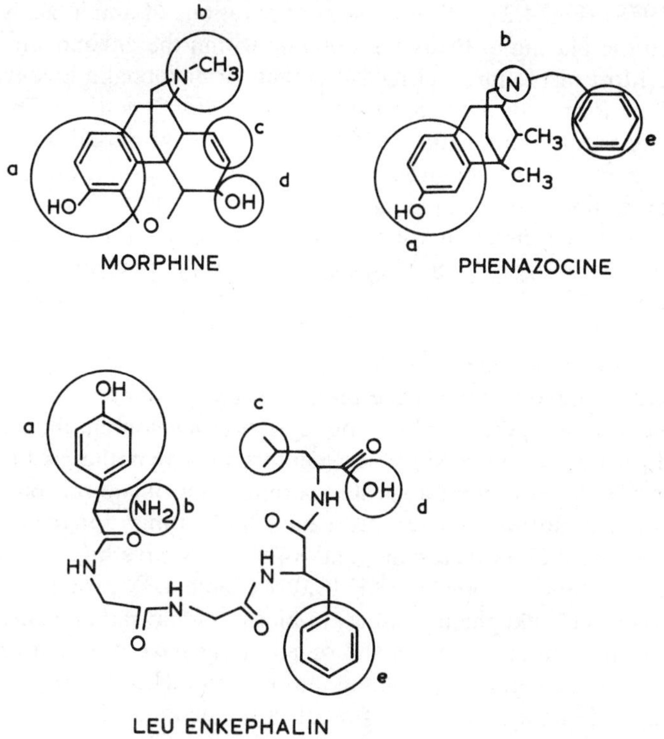

MORPHINE   PHENAZOCINE

LEU ENKEPHALIN

Fig. 4.2 Common structural features of opiates and enkephalin, adapted from
the data of Smith and Griffin (1978). Features include: a, tyrosine phenol and
opiate ring A; b, tyrosine amino group and morphine N-methyl group; c,
C-terminal side chain and C_6–C_7 of morphine ring C; d, C-terminal carboxyl
group and morphine ring C hydroxyl; e, phenylalanine phenyl ring and
phenazocine ring F. Alternatively, the phenyl ring of phenylalanine could
correspond to C_7–C_8 of morphine ring C (Gorin *et al.*, 1978).

of tyrosine resembles tyramine, although an exact tyramine configuration
may not be necessary as long as the hydroxyl-to-amino group distance
remains fixed (Smith and Griffin, 1978; Gacel *et al.*, 1979). The role of the
two glycine residues may be to introduce a maximum degree of flexibility
to the molecule; i.e. hydrogen bonding can occur with a minimum of steric
hindrance from side chains in positions 2 and 3. The phenylalanine phenyl
ring may correspond to the F ring present in some opiates (phenazocine
but not morphine) (Smith and Griffin, 1978); alternatively, the phenyl ring
could approximate the C_5-C_6 carbon atoms of ring C in morphine (Gorin *et
al.*, 1978). The C-terminal methionine or leucine side chain could
correspond to the C_6-C_7 region on ring C while the terminal carboxyl
group may correspond to the C_6 hydroxyl group of morphine (Smith and

Neurotransmitter Receptors

Griffin, 1978) (Fig. 4.2). All of these configurations of amino acids 2–5 depend on the placing of hydrogen bonding within the enkephalin molecule. Most of the physical measurements of enkephalin in solution and in crystalline form indicate some kind of β-turn (Jones *et al.*, 1976; Roques *et al.*, 1976; Smith and Griffin, 1978). Many of the proposed hydrogen bonding schemes do not fit structure–activity data (Gorin *et al.*, 1978), but these data do not rule out binding between the carbonyl of tyr and amino of gly_3, or between the amino of tyr and the carbonyl of gly_3, or even models incorporating hydrogen bonding between the first three residues of enkephalin.

(b) Multiple opiate receptors

The structure–activity studies have brought renewed interest in the concept that the central and peripheral nervous systems may contain different classes of opiate receptors. Multiple receptors were hypothesized in brain by Martin (1976) with physiological experiments: μ-opiate receptors have high affinity for morphine, κ-receptors have high affinity for the mixed agonist-antagonist ketocyclazocine, and σ-receptors have high affinity for another mixed function opiate, SKF-10,047 (Table 4.3). Structure–activity studies of various enkephalin analogs in bioassays and radioreceptor assays have shown that opioid peptides and opiate drugs have different profiles in mouse vas deferens, guinea-pig ileum and rat brain (Lord *et al.*, 1977). In particular, while opiates are more potent in the ileum assay than

Table 4.3 Properties of multiple opiate receptors.

Receptor type	Physiological effect	Agonist	Representative tissue
μ	↓pulse ↓respiration ↓pain	morphine	ileum brain (^{3}H-dihydromorphine)
κ	↓pain no effect: pulse and respiration	ketocyclazocine	ileum brain (^{3}H-ethylketocyclazocine)
σ	↑pulse ↑respiration ↓pain	SKF 10,047	brain (^{3}H-SKF 10,047)
δ	unknown	enkephalin	vas deferens, brain (^{3}H-enkephalin)

Data are from Martin *et al.* (1976) and Lord *et al.* (1977) and represent a partial summary of the physiological studies.

enkephalins, the reverse is true for the vas deferens. Moreover, while naloxone is equipotent in antagonizing opiates and enkephalin in the ileum, it is much less potent in antagonizing enkephalin than the opiates in the vas deferens. β-endorphin, on the other hand, is equipotent in the ileum and vas deferens. Detailed studies of the potency profile of a number of analogs and drugs suggest that receptors in the ileum closely resemble μ-receptors while those in the vas deferens represent a new class, δ-receptors, with high affinity for peptides and low affinity for opiate alkaloids. These results were extended by Shaw and Turnbull (1978) with a series of analogs in which gly_2 was substituted with D-amino acids, and by Lemaire *et al.* (1978a) with a series of D-ala-β-endorphin analogs to show that changes in the structure of these peptides had differential effects on potency in both the ileum and vas deferens assays. Such data are consistent with the idea that the two peripheral systems contain different classes of opiate receptor.

The biochemical identification of multiple opiate receptors within the CNS has been a more complex question. The issue has mainly concerned the differences between ^{3}H-opiate and ^{3}H-enkephalin binding to brain membranes, and whether the 'enkephalin receptor' is different from the 'opiate receptor'. Chang and Cuatrecasas (1979b) observed different regional distributions for ^{125}I-D-ala-enkephalin and ^{3}H-dihydromorphine binding sites and interpreted differences as two classes of receptors. However, these data differed from other work which showed that the regional distribution of ^{3}H-met-enkephalin was indistinguishable from that of ^{3}H-opiates (Simantov *et al.*, 1977). Furthermore, recent *in vitro* autoradiography studies using various ^{3}H-ligands have revealed no significant differences in the neuroanatomical distribution of ^{3}H-D-ala-enkephalin, ^{3}H-dihydromorphine and ^{3}H-diprenorphine at the light microscopic level of resolution (S. Young and M. Kuhar, personal communication). Therefore, if multiple opiate receptors exist in the brain, they appear to have similar distributions as measured by present techniques.

Other studies have revealed that some opiate agonists (such as morphine) are weaker in displacing ^{3}H-enkephalin binding than in ^{3}H-opiate binding (Lord *et al.*, 1977; Chang and Cuatrecasas, 1979b; Childers *et al.*, 1979), but the interpretations are highly variable. Chang and Cuatrecasas hypothesized two classes of receptors: enkephalin receptors with high affinity for peptides and low affinity for opiates, and opiate receptors with approximately equal affinity for both opiates and enkephalin. Lord *et al.* (1977) had a similar conclusion and, analogous to the results in ileum and vas deferens, identified ^{3}H-dihydromorphine sites as μ-receptors, and ^{3}H-enkephalin sites as δ-receptors.

Another analysis (Childers *et al.*, 1979) was considerably different since it divided the opiate drugs into various categories according to their relative potencies in displacing ^{3}H-enkephalin and ^{3}H-opiate binding. For some drugs, such as etorphine, levorphanol, phenazocine, and the opioid peptides, the affinity of binding is the same, whether measured by competition with ^{3}H-met-enkephalin, ^{3}H-naloxone or ^{3}H-dihydromorphine. Other drugs, like morphine, oxymorphone, normorphine, and fentanyl, are 19 to 55 times more potent in competing for ^{3}H-dihydromorphine and ^{3}H-naloxone than for ^{3}H-met-enkephalin binding. One explanation for the differential affinities of these two groups of agonists is two classes of opiate receptors. Drugs with similar affinities for ^{3}H-enkephalin and for ^{3}H-opiate binding sites would bind to a true 'enkephalin receptor', while those drugs that are much less potent with ^{3}H-enkephalin binding would bind to a distinct 'opiate receptor'. Alternatively, one class of receptor may exist, and enkephalin may possess several points of attachment to the active site of the receptor. One such point may be the hydrophobic side chain of leucine or methionine in enkephalin, which may correspond to the C_6-C_7 region of ring C in opiates (Smith and Griffin, 1978). Drugs that contain hydrophobic moieties in this region are relatively potent in displacing ^{3}H-enkephalin. This model can be useful in predicting relative potencies of drugs by examining their C ring structure.

It is clear that at the present level of technology the issue of multiple opiate receptors in the brain is extremely complex and open to several lines of interpretation. Hopefully, the development of more specific ^{3}H-ligands, of better techniques for high-resolution neuroanatomical localization, and of irreversible drugs to block specific effects will help to clarify this crucial issue.

(c) β-endorphin

Given the fact that β-endorphin is six times larger than enkephalin, it is not surprising that the development of analogs and structure–activity studies are further advanced for enkephalin than for β-endorphin. However, recent studies have analysed the activities of a large series of β-LPH products to determine what portions of the β-endorphin molecule are required for biological activity. Of primary importance, of course, is the 5 *N*-terminal amino acids corresponding to the sequence of met-enkephalin, without any one of which β-endorphin loses all opioid activity (Li *et al.*, 1978b). Starting with met-enkephalin as the core peptide, Yeung *et al.* (1978) added one amino acid at a time until the entire sequence of β-endorphin was obtained. Extension of enkephalin leads to a decline in activity until at least residue 17, when activity begins to rise above that of enkephalin. The activity does not approach that of β-endorphin until at least residue 29, thus indicating that practically the entire sequence of β-endorphin is required for full activity as measured by the ileum. Analgesia is even more stringent:

β-endorphin$_{1-30}$ has only 56 per cent of the analgesic (i.c.v.) potency as the parent molecule (Li *et al.*, 1978a). It is not known whether the addition of the non-enkephalin segment up to residue 31 is necessary for folding the enkephalin sequence in the proper conformation for the receptor active site, or whether the non-enkephalin segment has its own binding sites on or near the opiate receptor. Alternatively, the entire non-enkephalin segment may simply be required to protect the enkephalin sequence from proteolysis.

Analogous to D-ala$_2$-enkephalin, various D-amino acids have been incorporated into β-endorphin. Although D-amino acids in residues other than residue 2 result in decreased potency (Yamashiro *et al.*, 1978), D-ala$_2$-β-endorphin displays increased potency in analgesia tests (Walker *et al.*, 1977) and in vas deferens assay (Lemaire *et al.*, 1978a). However, the relative increase in potency of D-ala-β-endorphin compared to β-endorphin is not nearly as great as the increased potency of D-ala-enkephalin compared to enkephalin.

4.4.4 Irreversible opiate receptor ligands

All conventional opiate alkaloids and peptides are reversible ligands. The development of ligands that bind covalently to the active site of the opiate receptor would be a great benefit in addressing several problems: the solubilization and isolation of opiate receptors, the measurement of receptor turnover rate, and the determination of physiological roles for opiate receptors in animals whose receptors had been irreversibly blocked.

One method of using reversible ligands instead of irreversible drugs is to choose those ligands whose dissociation rates are relatively slow. The slowest dissociating opiates include etorphine, diprenorphine and enkephalin (Simantov *et al.*, 1978). Thus, etorphine has been used in attempts to solubilize receptors (Simon *et al.*, 1975a), while ^{3}H-diprenorphine has been used to label opiate receptors *in vivo* for autoradiography (Pert *et al.*, 1976b). The obvious difficulty with such ligands is that although they are slow to dissociate, they are eventually removed and the label is lost.

A more useful approach is to synthesize a new opiate which would covalently interact with the active site. One such method is to attach an alkylating agent to a potent opiate drug. Recently, Portoghese *et al.* (1978) synthesized chlornaltrexamine, an alkylating derivative of the antagonist naltrexone (Fig. 4.3). The molecule consists of an alkylating group, *bis* (α-chloroethyl) amine, attached to the C ring of naltrexone. Intracerebral injections of the drug produced blockade of morphine analgesia which lasted 3 days. Further, chlornaltrexamine addition to membranes *in vitro* blocked ^{3}H-naloxone binding through several washes, suggesting that chlornaltrexamine irreversibly blocked opiate receptor sites. Attachment of the same alkylating group to the corresponding agonist oxymorphone led to

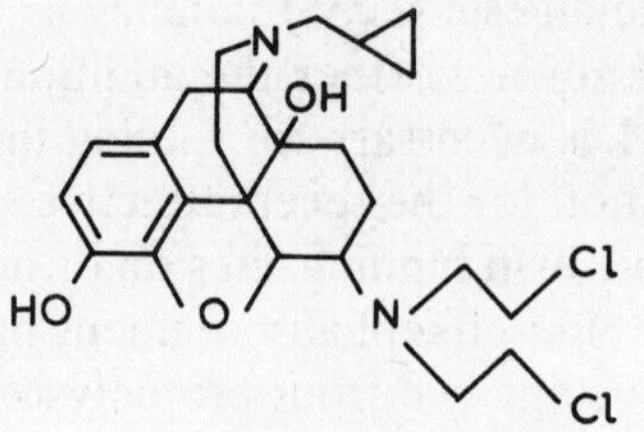

CHLORNALTREXAMINE 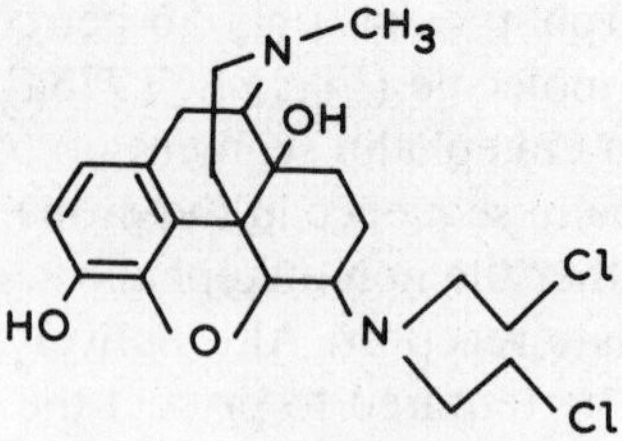   CHLOROXYMORPHAMINE

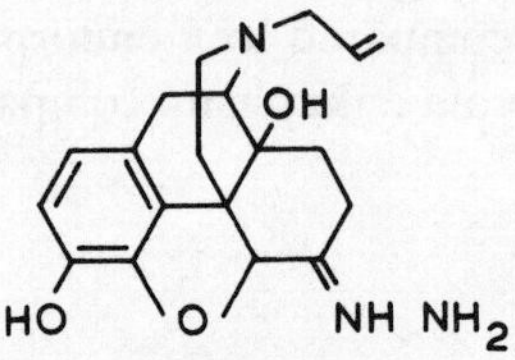

NALOXAZONE

Fig. 4.3 Structures of irreversible opiate drugs.

the formation of chloroxymorphamine (Fig. 4.3). In the ileum assay, chloroxymorphamine irreversibly inhibited electrically induced contractions. Naloxone failed to reverse the inhibition if added after chloroxymorphamine, but pretreatment of ileum with naloxone completely prevented the actions of the alkylating agonist (Caruso *et al.*, 1979). Since both agonist and antagonist alkylating drugs were effective at low concentrations, these agents may be valuable tools in receptor isolation studies.

Another irreversible opiate has been prepared by attaching a hydrazone moiety to naloxone, resulting in naloxazone (Fig. 4.3) (Pasternak *et al.*, 1980). Naloxazone blocked morphine analgesia in mice at least 24 h after subcutaneous injection. One day after naloxazone administration, high-affinity ^{3}H-naloxone binding in mouse brain was abolished, while low-affinity binding was not affected, indicating that only high-affinity opiate receptors mediate analgesia. Therefore, naloxazone can be used to differentiate the pharmacological properties of high- and low-affinity sites. Preliminary data indicate that 24 h after naloxazone injection, mice whose morphine analgesia had been blocked were not protected against lethal doses of morphine, suggesting analgesia and morphine lethality may be mediated by different classes of receptor.

An indirect method of irreversibly labeling receptor sites is to utilize non-specific alkylating agents to label all sites except those which have been protected by pretreatment with specific opiates. For example, Loh *et al.* (1976) used ^{125}I-iododiazosulfanilic acid (DISA) to bind to cerebroside sulfate moieties near the active site of the opiate receptor. Membranes were treated with unlabeled DISA in the presence of opiate isomers. After removal of the opiates, the membranes were incubated with ^{125}I-DISA; cerebroside sulfate was labeled only in preparations containing active stereoisomers. Another useful agent could be phenoxybenzamine, normally considered an adrenergic alkylating agent but which blocks opiate receptors at concentrations of about 1 μM (Spiehler *et al.*, 1978).

4.5 ENKEPHALIN AND β-ENDORPHIN AS NEUROTRANSMITTERS

Can opioid peptides be classified as true neurotransmitters? The criteria for answering such a question include: synthesis within specific neurons, storage and release from synaptic vesicles, interactions with post- or pre-synaptic receptors (including evidence of electrophysiological actions on neuronal firing rates), a mechanism for rapid termination of action by degradation or re-uptake, presence of discrete neuronal pathways, and behavioral or physiological reactions to the proposed neurotransmitter to indicate direct CNS actions. This section will deal with each criterion separately to help determine the neuronal identity of enkephalin and β-endorphin.

4.5.1 Subcellular and anatomical distribution of enkephalin and β-endorphin

A critical question concerning the neuronal roles of the opioid peptides is whether they are distributed evenly inside neurons or whether they are stored within discrete vesicles. Subcellular fractionation studies have shown that opioid activity in rat brain is enriched in synaptosomal fractions (Simantov *et al.*, 1976b), and in bovine brain and pituitary it is enriched in cytoplasmic granule fractions (Queen *et al.*, 1976). However, like all biochemical fractionations, contamination of other subcellular elements remains a problem. More resolution has been obtained in an electron microscopic study of enkephalin immunoactivity in rat brain (Pickel *et al.*, 1979). Visualized by peroxidase–antiperoxidase immunocytochemical techniques, enkephalin was localized to axon terminals inside several large dense vesicles and outside the rim of many small clear vesicles. The enkephalinergic terminals formed asymmetric synaptic junctions with dendrites containing tyrosine hydroxylase.

If enkephalin is stored in vesicles like typical neurotransmitters, the enkephalinergic neuronal pathways should be identified in specific areas of the brain. Immunohistochemical mapping of brain areas with enkephalin antisera have provided a high-resolution picture of the neuroanatomical distribution of enkephalin; details of these studies have been reviewed elsewhere (Uhl *et al.*, 1978a). The identification of specific enkephalinergic pathways has been accomplished by performing specific lesions. For example, injection of kainic acid (a glutamic acid analog that destroys cell bodies around the site of injection) into rat striatum reduced striatum levels of enkephalin by 50 per cent (Hong *et al.*, 1977; Childers *et al.*, 1978), suggesting that half of striatal enkephalin is present in neurons intrinsic to the striatum. Cuello and Paxinos (1978) found that cutting the boundary between the caudate and globus pallidus reduced enkephalin immunofluorescence in the globus, indicating that enkephalinergic cell bodies in the caudate project axons into the globus pallidus. However, this interpretation may be doubtful since extensive electrolytic lesions in the caudate had no effect on enkephalin fluorescence in the globus pallidus (R. Innis and F. Correa, personal communication), suggesting that the knife-cut lesions of the previous study could have destroyed globus neurons. Another enkephalinergic pathway has been located projecting from the central amygdaloid nucleus to the stria terminalis by observing a decrease of enkephalin immunofluorescence in stria terminalis following lesions of the amygdala (Uhl *et al.*, 1978b). In the spinal cord, enkephalin is largely confined to small interneurons in the dorsal gray since dorsal rhizotomy and hemisections fail to decrease enkephalin immunofluorescence. Lesions of the paraventricular nucleus of the hypothalamus decrease enkephalin immunofluorescence in the median eminence, indicating a pathway from the paraventricular neucleus to the median eminence (Hokfelt *et al.*, 1977). Other lesions of the paraventricular nucleus reduce enkephalin levels in the neurointermediate lobe of the pituitary (Rossier *et al.*, 1979), suggesting that pituitary enkephalin occurs in fibers which project from the hypothalamus. Therefore, all of the lesion and nonlesioned studies picture enkephalin as a peptide that is widely distributed in brain in discrete pathways.

Recent studies have focused on the distribution of β-endorphin and β-LPH in the CNS (Bloom *et al.*, 1978; Watson *et al.*, 1978). Unlike the wide distribution of enkephalin, the neuronal pathways for β-endorphin are very limited. The main β-endorphin pathway consists of a single hypothalamic cell group with long ascending projections to the ventral spetum, nucleus accumbens and the paraventricular nucleus of the thalamus, and long descending fibers into the brain stem (especially the periaqueductal gray, locus coeruleus and reticular formation). Radioimmunoassays confirm the different distribution of β-endorphin and enkephalin; although the hypothalamus contains high levels of both peptides, other areas (such as

caudate and the globus pallidus) contain much more enkephalin than
β-endorphin (Krieger *et al.*, 1977; Rossier *et al.*, 1977b; Bloom *et al.*, 1978).
Perhaps the most dramatic example is the spinal cord, which contains high
levels of enkephalin in Laminae I and II but is almost completely deficient
in β-endorphin. Even in the hypothalamus, enkephalin and β-endorphin
have different distributions: Watson *et al.* (1978) stained serial sections of
rat hypothalamus and although β-endorphin, β-LPH and ACTH were
present in the same cells, enkephalin did not overlap into any of the
β-endorphin cells. The same study revealed that lesions of the basal
hypothalamus to destroy β-endorphin caused large decreases in β-LPH but
no effect in enkephalin levels in both anterior and posterior sections of the
brain. These experiments clearly point out that, despite their structural
similarities, enkephalin and β-endorphin represent two separate neuronal
systems.

4.5.2 Biosynthesis

The first goal of biosynthesis studies is to determine whether the
brain-opioid peptides are synthesized within the CNS or arise from other
sources. Since hypophysectomy has no effect on brain levels of enkephalin
(Cheung and Goldstein, 1976) or β-endorphin (Rossier *et al.*, 1977b), the
brain peptides are not derived from pituitary endorphins. Intracerebral
injections of protein synthesis inhibitors such as cycloheximide and puromycin
reduced brain levels of met- and leu-enkephalin (Gros *et al.*, 1978; Childers
and Snyder, 1979a), suggesting that enkephalin may be formed by normal
protein synthesis mechanisms in the brain. Infusion of labeled amino acids
into rat ventricles and isolation of labeled peptides by met-enkephalin
antibody affinity columns yielded a significant (though small) quantity of
labeled enkephalin (Yang *et al.*, 1978b). These results provide the most
direct evidence that enkephalin is synthesized within the brain. Similarly,
enkephalin synthesis in intestine has been detected by incubating ileum
slices with labeled amino acids (Sosa *et al.*, 1978).

If the synthesis of enkephalin and β-endorphin does occur in the brain,
another important question is whether they are synthesized from high
molecular weight precursors. The identification of met-enkephalin as
residues 61–65 of β-LPH and of β-endorphin as $β\text{-LPH}_{61-91}$ led to the theory
that β-LPH is the precursor of both peptides. Although this is the case for
β-endorphin, the precursor relationships for enkephalin has not been as
clear.

The best evidence of β-endorphin precursors comes from the pituitary.
Early studies (Lazarus *et al.*, 1976) took advantage of the fact that β-LPH
has no opioid activity to show that incubations of β-LPH with pituitary
extracts results in the formation of opioid activity. Rubinstein *et al.* (1977)

have shown that storage of fresh pituitaries increases levels of β-endorphin, suggesting endogenous formation of precursors. The pituitary precursor was identified in an elegant series of experiments by Mains *et al.* (1977), who demonstrated that ACTH and β-endorphin share a common precursor, a 30 000 molecular weight protein known as 'Big ACTH', or recently renamed pro-opiocortin (Rubinstein *et al.*, 1978). In pituitary tumor cell lines, sequential immunoprecipitation of 'Big ACTH' with ACTH and β-endorphin antisera revealed that both antisera precipitated the same protein. Further, trypsin digests of 'Big ACTH' yielded peptides similar in structure to β-LPH and β-endorphin as well as ACTH (Mains *et al.*, 1977). Identical results were obtained in rat pituitary extracts (Rubinstein *et al.*, 1978) and in intact toad pituitaries (Loh, 1979). These findings were confirmed by a different technique (Crine *et al.*, 1977, 1978) with synthesis of labeled β-endorphin from β-LPH and the ACTH/β-LPH precursor with pulse-label experiments in rat pars intermedia. The precursor molecule also reacts with α-MSH and β-MSH antisera (Mains *et al.*, 1977; Loh, 1979), suggesting that the ACTH/β-LPH precursor may contain a variety of hormones.

A remarkable amount of information about the ACTH/β-LPH precursor has been obtained from cell-free systems in which the precursor has been synthesized *in vitro* from mRNA. Roberts and Herbert (1977) isolated mRNA from pituitary tumor cells and showed that β-LPH tryptic peptides are located on the C-terminal side of ACTH tryptic peptides. Even more details were obtained by Nakanishi *et al.* (1978, 1979) who isolated the DNA which codes for the ACTH/β-LPH precursor. After isolation of mRNA from bovine pituitaries and verifying the cell-free protein product as the precursor (Nakanishi *et al.*, 1979), the DNA was synthesized *in vitro* from mRNA by reverse transcription. The DNA was inserted into a bacterial plasmid, then cloned, isolated and sequenced. The 1091-base pair DNA product therefore described the exact theoretical amino acid sequence of the entire ACTH/β-LPH precursor and allowed construction of a complete map of the molecule (Fig. 4.4). The map shows a protein of molecular weight 29 259 with several repeating features: MSH-like peptides are present at least three times (α-, β- and γ-MSH, the latter previously unidentified but discovered by analysis of the nucleotide sequence) and ACTH$_{4-10}$ is present in the sequence of β-LPH. Such repetitions of peptide sequences, coupled with an unusually high C + G nucleotide base content and several nucleotide base duplications, have led Nakanishi *et al.* (1979) to suggest that the ACTH/β-LPH precursor could have evolved through a series of gene duplications.

The next challenge for the study of the pituitary ACTH/β-LPH precursor is to determine how the molecule is broken down into active hormones and how such a process is regulated. The map of the precursor (Fig. 4.4) reveals

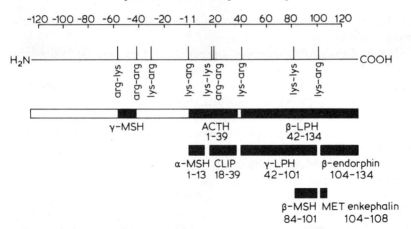

Fig. 4.4 Map of pituitary ACTH/β-LPH precursor protein, adapted from Nakanishi *et al.* (1979). Top numbers represent amino acid residues with residue 1 of ACTH being residue + 1 of the precursor; residue − 131 is considered as the *N*-terminus. Vertical lines represent paired basic amino acid residues; note that all biologically active peptides (depicted below the precursor as shaded areas) are bracketted by such residues with the exception of met-enkephalin.

that each active peptide is bracketted by pairs of basic amino acid residues; i.e. lys-lys, arg-arg, or lys-arg. Such pairs are extremely susceptible to the actions of trypsin-like enzymes which are present in pituitary (Bradbury *et al.*, 1976c) and which may activate the peptides. The regulation of hydrolysis of the precursor could be accomplished by post-translational additions to the molecule. For example, the ACTH/β-LPH precursor is a glyco-protein (Loh, 1979) and inhibition of glycosylation by tunicamycin causes rapid degradation of the precursor and formation of atypical peptides (Loh and Gainer, 1978). Thus, glycosylation of the precursor may protect it from non-specific hydrolysis. Smyth *et al.* (1979) have demonstrated the formation of *N*-acetyl β-endorphin in pituitary. *N*-acetylation of β-endorphin causes a loss of activity in opiate binding preparations and may represent a mechanism in which certain specific products of the precursor could be inactivated.

Studies of the mechanism of synthesis of β-endorphin in brain are not nearly as advanced as those in pituitary. As mentioned previously, immunohistochemical studies have revealed that cells and fibers that stain for β-endorphin and β-LPH also stain for ACTH (Bloom *et al.*, 1978), indicating that the ACTH/β-LPH precursor may exist in brain as well as pituitary. Direct evidence was obtained by Liotta *et al.* (1979), who used sequential immunoprecipitation of labeled proteins in cultured hypothalamus cells to show β-endorphin and ACTH determinants in the same protein(s).

Whether β-endorphin serves as a precursor for enkephalin in the brain is the subject of much investigation. Incubation of brain slices with β-endorphin results in the formation of met-enkephalin (Austen and Smyth, 1977; Aono *et al.*, 1978). But whether this conversion takes place physiologically is questionable. First, brain levels of β-endorphin are only 5 to 10 per cent those of enkephalin (Rossier *et al.*, 1977b; Simantov *et al.*, 1977). Moreover, as discussed earlier, the regional localizations of β-endorphin and enkephalin throughout the brain differ considerably.

Other attempts to identify enkephalin precursors in brain have searched for high molecular weight proteins that contain the enkephalin sequence and therefore cross-react with enkephalin antibodies. One study (Childers and Snyder, 1979b) showed that soluble rat brain proteins contain two peaks of enkephalin immunoreactivity, one of which reacts non-specifically with immunoglobulins and a second (40 000 to 60 000 molecular weight) which is more specific. Digestion of the second peak by trypsin results in the formation of a smaller polypeptide (1000 to 2000 molecular weight), which possesses both enkephalin-like immunoreactivity and opioid activity but which is not identical to enkephalin, indicating that trypsin is not the endogenous enkephalin-forming enzyme in the brain. Similar results from other groups (Lewis *et al.*, 1978; Yang *et al.*, 1978a) support the idea that high molecular weight precursors of enkephalin exist in brain. Recently, Kangawa *et al.*, (1979) confirmed the existence in brain of a 15-amino acid peptide which contains the sequence of leu-enkephalin. Called 'α-neo-endorphin', the peptide has the sequence tyr-gly-gly-phe-leu-arg-lys-arg-(pro, gly, tyr, lys_2, arg) which suggests the possible formation of leu–enkephalin by trypsin-like enzymes. The peptide has six times the activity of enkephalin in the guinea-pig ileum bioassay. Since the structure of α-neo-endorphin is different from that of β-endorphin, it provides further evidence against the role of β-endorphin as precursor of enkephalin, and represents the first identification of larger peptides in brain containing the sequence of leu-enkephalin.

4.5.3 Release and degradation

A key requirement for the actions of a neurotransmitter is demonstration of its release from presynaptic nerve endings. Calcium-dependent release of enkephalin has been reported from rat brain synaptosomes (Smith *et al.*, 1976) and from striatum (Henderson *et al.*, 1978; Osborne *et al.*, 1978) and globus pallidus slices (Iversen *et al.*, 1978). Release of enkephalin may also occur in peripheral neurons. Puig *et al.* (1977) studied release of opiate-like activity in the guinea-pig ileum. In this system, stimulation of ileum at a high frequency results in inhibition of electrically stimulated contraction, an effect similar to that of exogenous opiates or enkephalins. This effect is reversed by opiate antagonists in a stereospecific manner, and release is calcium-dependent (Oka and Sawa, 1979). Another study (Schulz *et al.*, 1977) utilized a specific radioimmunoassay for enkephalin to demonstrate that enkephalin itself is released from isolated strips of guinea-pig ileum following electrical stimulation.

After a neurotransmitter is released and binds to its specific receptor its actions must be rapidly terminated, normally by active re-uptake into pre-synaptic terminals or degradation by specific enzyme systems. So far, experiments have failed to detect significant active uptake of ^{3}H-D-ala–enkephalin into brain synaptosomes at 37° C when such uptake is carefully differentiated from endogenous receptor binding (Osborne *et al.*, 1978; S.R. Childers and S.H. Snyder, unpublished data). Therefore, most studies have focused on the possibility that the brain contains a specific 'enkephalinase' to degrade the peptides.

As mentioned earlier, enkephalin is extremely susceptible to proteolysis. In fact, non-specific aminopeptidases can inactivate enkephalin so rapidly (by splitting off the N-terminal tyrosine) that the necessity for a specific enkephalinase for effective degradation seemed doubtful. However, recent evidence from Schwartz's group (Malfroy *et al.*, 1978) indicates that a dipeptidase with high affinity for enkephalin exists in mouse striatum membranes. The enzyme splits between the gly_3 and phe_4 bond of both met- and leu-enkephalin and therefore is not an aminopeptidase. The enzyme had a K_m of approximately 1 μM for enkephalin as well as D-ala-enkephalin, β-endorphin, substance P and a variety of other peptides. The dipeptidase also acts on several compounds (e.g. bradykinin and hip-his-leu) which are substrates for angiotensin-converting enzymes, but is less active against other such inhibitors, suggesting that 'enkephalinase' is similar but not identical to angiotensin-converting enzyme (Swerts *et al.*, 1979). The lack of specificity of the dipeptidase may indicate the absence of a highly specific 'enkephalinase'. Nevertheless, the fact that the regional distribution of 'enkephalinase' and effects of lesions (kainic acid injection into striatum and 6-hydroxydopamine lesion of the nigrostriatal pathway) on 'enkephalinase' activity paralleled those of opiate receptors and of enkephalin itself suggests that the enzyme may be specific for enkephalin (Malfroy *et al.*, 1979). One exciting possibility is the role of enkephalinase in opiate addiction: in morphine-dependent rats, 'enkephalinase' activity was increased by 59 per cent with no effect on amino peptidases (Malfroy *et al.*, 1978). These results suggest that during chronic morphine treatment, neurons may increase enkephalinase in an attempt to restore the activity of the endogenous opioid system to normal levels. Thus, morphine abstinence might cause withdrawal symptoms because increased enkephalinase would degrade released enkephalin resulting in a loss of function of the endogenous opioid system.

4.5.4 Interactions with other neurotransmitter systems

The discovery of presynaptic opiate receptors in the brain and spinal cord (Lamotte *et al.*, 1976; Atweh *et al.*, 1978; Childers *et al.*, 1978) suggests that opiate receptors and their endogenous ligands may exert their actions by modulating the release of other neurotransmitters. The most convincing evidence so far for such interactions involve substance P and the catecholamines.

Enkephalin and substance P appear to interact in the spinal cord, where opiate receptors are present on sensory afferents and enkephalin is located in small interneurons. Presynaptic inhibition of the release of the excitatory sensory transmitter by enkephalin could explain analgesic effects at the spinal level. A strong candidate for the 'pain' sensory transmitter whose release would be inhibited by enkephalin is substance P. Opiates selectively block release of substance P from slices of the substantia gelatinosa of the trigeminal (Jessell and Iversen, 1977). D-ala–enkephalin inhibits potassium-induced release of substance P from cultured sensory neurons (Mudge *et al.*, 1979); however, this effect occurs only at high concentrations (10 μM) of D-ala-enkephalin.

Much evidence has accumulated to suggest an involvement of enkephalin with catecholamine systems. The electron microscopic study of Pickel *et al.* (1979) clearly showed that in the locus coeruleus, axon terminals which contain enkephalin formed synapses with dendrites that stain for tyrosine hydroxylase. Therefore, a direct anatomical connection exists between enkephalin and catecholamine neurons. Biochemical experiments have also suggested a relationship. In mouse vas deferens, for example, enkephalin blocks the potassium-stimulated release of norepinephrine (Henderson, 1976). Enkephalin (Taube *et al.*, 1976) and β-endorphin (Arbilla and Langer, 1978) block stimulated release of norepinephrine from cerebral cortex. These effects of enkephalin and β-endorphin can be reversed by naloxone, suggesting that presynaptic opiate receptors are present on noradrenergic nerve terminals. The relation between opioid peptides and dopamine is less clear. Loh *et al.* (1976) demonstrated that β-endorphin inhibited the potassium-induced release of dopamine in rat striatum; these results, however, have not been confirmed (Arbilla and Langer, 1978).

Interaction of opioid peptides and catecholamines helps to explain some behavioral effects of the peptides. For example, intracerebral injection of β-endorphin causes catalepsy (Bloom *et al.*, 1976; Jacquet and Marks, 1976), which is consistent with the idea that opiates inhibit dopamine release in the caudate. Another type of evidence was provided by Pollard *et al.* (1977) who showed that lesions of the nigro-striatal pathway by 6-hydroxydopamine decreased opiate receptor binding in the striatum, suggesting the presence of presynaptic opiate receptors on dopaminergic terminals. In addition, α-adrenergic binding was increased in morphine-dependent rats (Pollard *et al.*, 1977), so that addiction could cause a chronic inhibition of catecholamine release which would result in a compensatory increase in the number of catecholamine receptors.

The mechanism of action of enkephalin on neuronal systems has been studied by electrophysiological experiments. In general, the actions of microiontophoretically applied enkephalin are inhibitory; two exceptions are naloxone-reversible excitations in Renshaw cells in the spinal cord (Davies and Dray, 1976) and pyramidal cells in the hippocampus (Nicoll *et al.*, 1977). A recent study of the hippocampus (Fry *et al.*, 1979) revealed that excitatory responses to enkephalin are not reversed by naloxone and are not stereospecific, indicating that such responses are non-specific whereas inhibitory effects of opiates generally are specific. Naloxone-reversible depression of neuronal firing by enkephalins has been observed in the cerebral cortex (Fredrickson and Norris, 1976; Hill *et al.*, 1976; Zieglgansberger and Frey, 1976), thalamus (Hill *et al.*, 1976), caudate (Fredrickson and Norris, 1976; Hill *et al.*, 1976; Zieglgansberger and Frey, 1976), periaqueductal grey (Fredrickson and Norris, 1976), brainstem (Bradley *et al.*, 1976), and spinal cord (Duggan *et al.*, 1976; Zieglgansberger and Frey, 1976). In thalamus, neurons that are stimulated by noxious stimuli are also depressed by enkephalin (Hill *et al.*, 1976). In addition, neurons in the myenteric plexus of guinea-pig ileum are depressed by enkephalin (North and Williams, 1976).

The electrophysiological experiments have generated some debate concerning the mechanism of action of enkephalin. Since enkephalin abolishes glutamate-induced activity in some regions, its major action may be on postsynaptic receptors (Gent and Wolstencroft, 1976; Zieglgansberger and Bayerl, 1976). Zieglgansberger and Frey (1976) showed that in spinal cord, enkephalin-induced depression occurs without hyperpolarization (with no detectable effect on either membrane resting potential or on membrane resistance) and suggested that enkephalin may block the actions of excitatory transmitters in opening sodium channels. However, in mouse spinal cell culture (Macdonald and Nelson, 1978) opiates reduce the quantal content of excitatory postsynaptic potentials and not their size, indicating a presynaptic action of opiates. A recent study of enkephalin-inhibited spinal neurons in the cat (Zieglgansberger and Tulloch, 1979) provides a model of both pre- and postsynaptic enkephalinergic contacts in the spinal cord to decrease the efficacy of excitatory neurotransmitters.

4.5.5 Analgesia and behavior

In general, many of the physiological roles of neurotransmitters should relate ultimately to some form of behavior. In the particular case of the opioid peptides, at least part of the function should concern analgesia. A number of studies have attempted to show that opioid peptides are natural analgesics; i.e. neurotransmitters released by specific neurons in various pain-mediating pathways. Enkephalin itself is a weak analgesic, effective only when injected intraventricularly or directly into the periaqueductal grey (Belluzzi *et al.*, 1976; Buscher *et al.*, 1976; Chang *et al.*, 1976). However, the effective intracerebral dose of D-ala-met-enkephalin is considerably lower and the duration of action is longer than that of met-enkephalin, suggesting that the weak potency of enkephalin is due to rapid degradation in the brain (Pert, 1976; Dutta *et al.*, 1977; Wei *et al.*, 1977). In addition, D-ala-enkephalin is effective when administered intravenously (Dutta *et al.*, 1977). An even more effective analgesic is the synthetic enkephalin analog FK-33-824, which is 30 000 and 1 000 times more potent than met-enkephalin and morphine, respectively, after intracerebral administration (Roemer *et al.*, 1977). It is also effective by subcutaneous and oral administration. Other enkephalin analogs which are resistant to proteolysis are also effective analgesics; their potencies are summarized in Table 4.1. β-endorphin itself is an effective intravenous analgesic and is over 1000 times more potent than met-enkephalin when given intracerebrally (Bradbury *et al.*, 1976a; Graf *et al.*, 1976; Loh *et al.*, 1976; Tseng, *et al.*, 1976; Wei *et al.*, 1977). However, β-endorphin is less active than FK-33-824 in intracerebral injections (Roemer *et al.*, 1977).

Repeated administration of either enkephalin or β-endorphin results in the development of tolerance (Chang *et al.*, 1976; Van Ree *et al.*, 1976; Waterfield *et al.*, 1976) as well as physical dependence as measured by self-administration studies (Belluzzi *et al.*, 1976; Van Ree *et al.*, 1979). Tolerance to the analgesic actions of β-endorphin can even occur following a single i.c.v. dose of the peptide (Huidrobro-Toro and Way, 1978).

Other evidence has associated the opioid peptides with an endogenous analgesic system. As previously mentioned, electrophysiological experiments in the spinal cord have demonstrated specific enkephalin inhibition of nociceptive neurons (Hill *et al.*, 1976). The development of stimulation analgesia (Reynolds, 1969; Mayer and Liebeskind, 1974) suggested the release of endogenous analgesics, a proposal that is supported by an increase in immunoreactive β-endorphin in the ventricular fluid of patients being stimulated in the periaqueductal grey (Hosobuchi *et al.*, 1979). These issues are discussed in more detail by Terenius (1978).

The opioid peptides, particularly β-endorphin, also cause profound behavioral changes when injected intracerebrally. Perhaps the most common behavioral change is the development of muscular rigidity and immobility which lasts several hours (Segal *et al.*, 1977). Other behavioral changes include catalepsy (Bloom *et al.*, 1976; Jacquet and Marks, 1976), hyperactivity (Segal *et al.*, 1977; Wei *et al.*, 1977), seizures (Urca *et al.*, 1977), sedation (Jacquet and Marks, 1976) and control of appetite (Margules *et al.*, 1978). All effects can be reversed by naloxone. β-endorphin is much more potent than met- or leu-enkephalin, and slightly more potent than D-ala-enkephalin (Wei *et al.*, 1977). There is some evidence that enkephalin analogs provide qualitatively different behavioral reactions from β-endorphin; for example, enkephalin analogs may produce hyperactivity more often than β-endorphin (Wei *et al.*, 1977).

An intriguing effect has been reported by DeWied *et al.* (1978) from studies with γ-endorphin (β-LPH$_{61-77}$). This peptide, although fairly potent in opiate assays, has effects opposite from β-endorphin and enkephalin in extinction of pole-jumping behavior. Removal of tyr$_1$, yielding des-tyr-γ-endorphin, predictably destroys opioid activity. However, des-tyr-γ-endorphin possesses other behavioral effects, in particular neuroleptic-type actions to facilitate pole-jumping avoidance, reduce passive avoidance and facilitate 'grip tests'. Haloperidol parallels these actions on rats. These results suggest that des-tyr-γ-endorphin (or some related peptide) may act as an endogenous neuroleptic, and raise the interesting possibility that, if changes of one amino acid in a peptide can completely alter its behavioral effects then genetic errors in peptide synthesis or metabolism can play an important role in the development of abnormal behavioral states. This important discovery must be confirmed and extended; in the meantime, however, Pedigo *et al.* (1979) recently demonstrated that des-tyr-γ-endorphin did not displace ^{3}H-haloperidol binding in brain membranes, indicating that the neuroleptic actions of the peptide must involve sites other than dopamine receptors. The apparent neuroleptic effects of des-tyr-γ-endorphin on rats have prompted clinical studies in schizophrenic patients. In double-blind, cross-over experimental designs, low doses of this peptide markedly improved schizophrenic patients (Verhoeven *et al.*, 1979).

4.6 OPIOID PEPTIDES IN PERIPHERAL TISSUES

Although most attention has been focused on CNS actions of opiates, both enkephalin and β-endorphin are present in peripheral tissues. In the pituitary, β-endorphin is the predominant opioid peptide (Rossier *et al.*, 1977b; Rubinstein *et al.*, 1977; Duka *et al.*, 1978). The highest concentration of β-endorphin in rat pituitary occurs in the pars intermedia, six times higher than that of the pars anterior and 30 times higher than that of

the pars nervosa (Duke *et al.*, 1978). Although preliminary studies indicated a complete lack of enkephalin in the pituitary, more recent results clearly
show that enkephalin is present in both anterior and posterior pituitary
(Rossier *et al.*, 1977b; Rubinstein *et al.*, 1977; Duka *et al.*, 1978), although
the amounts of enkephalin remain considerably low than β-endorphin.

One important question is what physiological roles the pituitary
β-endorphin could be playing. Clearly, a significant amount of pituitary
β-endorphin does not enter into the brain since levels of β-endorphin in
brains, measured by radioimmunoassay, are not altered by hypophysectomy.
β-endorphin may interact with opiate receptors in the pituitary, which were
described by Simantov and Snyder (1977). However, pituitary opiate
receptors are primarily localized to the posterior pituitary, an area which
contains relatively low levels of β-endorphin. Although some of the
β-endorphin in the pars intermedia may be released in such a way as to
interact with opiate receptors and influence secretion of vasopressin, most of
the β-endorphin probably performs other functions.

An endocrine function for β-endorphin was suggested by the finding that
β-endorphin and β-LPH are released along with ACTH into the
bloodstream following acute stress or glucocorticoid administration
(Guillemin, 1977b; Krieger *et al.*, 1977; Rossier *et al.*, 1977a). This
hypothesis was supported by Suda *et al.* (1978) who observed large increases
in plasma levels of β-endorphin and β-LPH in patients with endocrine
disorders (Cushing's disease and Nelson's syndrome) which result in
increased production of ACTH. It is not clear whether this secretion of
β-endorphin is the release of a physiologically important hormonal agent or
simply a coincidence of the fact that β-endorphin, β-LPH and ACTH are
produced from the same precursor and are stored within the same cells in
the pituitary. If β-endorphin is a circulating hormone, its principal target
organ has not yet been discovered. One possibility is that pituitary
β-endorphin may regulate the release of other pituitary hormones. It has
long been known that acute administration of opiate agonists have profound
effects on the regulation of pituitary hormone secretion. Recent studies have
shown that β-endorphin mimics the neuroendocrine effects of opiates: to
increase growth hormone (Cusan *et al.*, 1977), prolactin (Dupont *et al.*,
1977), leutinizing hormone (Takahara *et al.*, 1978), and α-MSH (Greidanus
et al., 1979), while decreasing TSH (Meites *et al.*, 1979) and vasopressin
(Greidanus *et al.*, 1979). These results must be viewed with caution since the
literature contains several contradictory reports; for example, studies of opioid
peptides which decreased leutinizing hormone (Meites *et al.*, 1979) and
increased vasopressin (Weitzman *et al.*, 1977). Whatever the final resolution
of these effects, however, it seems clear that circulating β-endorphin is not
the responsible agent. First, although all of the neuroendocrine effects of
β-endorphin can be reversed by naloxone and therefore involve some form

of opiate receptor, the effects are not restricted to β-endorphin but are matched by enkephalin as well (Cusan *et al.*, 1977; Shaar *et al.*, 1977; Meites *et al.*, 1979), which clearly is not a circulating hormone because of its susceptibility to serum proteases. Second, the actions of β-endorphin on pituitary may result from brain, not pituitary or circulating β-endorphin, since opiates or opioid peptides have no effect on hormone secretion from isolated anterior (Shaar *et al.*, 1977) or posterior (Weitzman *et al.*, 1977) pituitary cells. It appears more likely that opioid peptides affect neuroendocrine function from the hypothalamus (an area of the brain particularly rich in β-endorphin), perhaps by modulating activities of neurons carrying catecholamines or serotonin that regulate pituitary hormone release (Meites *et al.*, 1979).

If circulating β-endorphin has no direct effect on pituitary hormone release, an alternative role could be established as a possible circulating analgesic, suggested by the results of Pomeranz *et al.* (1977) who showed that hypophysectomy reduced the response of rats to acupuncture. These results are difficult to interpret since the probable outcome of analgesia mediated by circulating endorphins would be a generalized analgesia, not the localized analgesia seen in acupuncture (Terenius, 1978). Certainly, circulating β-endorphin has no effect on opiate tolerance and physical dependence (Holaday *et al.*, 1979), confirming that these effects are mediated by brain endorphins. Moreover, circulating levels of β-endorphin, 0.01 to 0.1 nM (Akil *et al.*, 1979), are much too low to attain analgesic concentration in the brain.

Still more possible functions for circulating β-endorphin have been explored by groups who measure physiological consequences of systemically administered β-endorphin. In one study, i.v. injections of β-endorphin produced prolonged hypotension in rats (Lemaire *et al.*, 1978b), although this effect may be a central action of β-endorphin since it is also seen when injected i.c.v. into dogs (Laubie *et al.*, 1977) and rats (Bolme *et al.*, 1978) and is blocked by treatment with serotonergic antagonists (Lemaire *et al.*, 1978b). One effect that does not involve CNS interactions was recently reported by Shanker and Sharma (1979): β-endorphin increased synthesis of corticosterone in isolated rat adrenal cells *in vitro*. Therefore, the adrenal cortex is a possible candidate for target organ of β-endorphin actions. The development of ^{3}H-β-endorphin preparations that are biologically active (Houghten and Ki, 1978) will hopefully reveal the existence of further peripheral β-endorphin receptors.

Enkephalin (and not β-endorphin) immunohistofluorescence has been reported in nerve fibers and cell bodies in sympathetic ganglia of rat and guinea-pig (Schultzberg *et al.*, 1979). Some cells (especially the 'small intensely fluorescent' cells) appear to contain both enkephalin immunoreactivity and norepinephrine. DiGuilio *et al.* (1979) have shown that enkephalin immunoreactivity in sympathetic ganglia is composed mostly of high molecular weight material with only a small quantity of enkephalin. A similar situation may exist in bovine adrenal medulla. Enkephalin immunofluorescence was discovered by Hokfelt's group (Schultzberg et al., 1978) in guinea-pig adrenal medulla endocrine cells. Characterization of this activity by gel filtration columns revealed several peaks of enkephalin immunoreactivity, at least one of which is larger than β-endorphin (Viveros et al., 1979; S.R. Childers and S.H. Snyder, unpublished results; E. Costa, personal communication). Enkephalin is stored in the chromaffin granules and secreted in a calcium-dependent release from granules with catecholamines after cholinergic stimulation (Viveros et al., 1979). Therefore, enkephalin is released from the adrenal gland under the same stimulus that releases catecholamines, although the possible role of the released enkephalin remains mysterious since the pentapeptides would immediately be destroyed by serum proteases. A critical unanswered question is the identification and role of the high molecular weight enkephalin-like activity in both adrenal medulla and sympathetic ganglia.

The existence of enkephalin in gut tissues has been known for several years. Indeed, enkephalin is one of a series of peptides found in brain and gut, including neurotensin, substance P, cholecystokinin and vasoactive intestinal peptides (Innis and Snyder, 1979). In the gastrointestinal tract, enkephalin immunofluorescence has been detected in fibers of the stomach, duodenum and rectum of guinea-pig (Miller and Cuatrecasas, 1978). In the guinea-pig ileum, enkephalin fibers appear mainly in Meissner's plexus and in the circular muscle layer. In the gut some studies indicate overlap of enkephalin immunofluorescence in the same endocrine cells that contain other peptides. Polak et al. (1977) found that endocrine cells of the central mucosa that stain for gastrin also stain for enkephalin. Similarly, in the pancreas, glucagon cells also contain enkephalin fluorescence (Grube et al., 1978). These results suggest that these peptides may share common precursors and if the experience cited above for adrenal medulla and sympathetic ganglia is any guide, point to the necessity of determining the biochemical identity of these immunoreactive products.

4.7 CONCLUDING REMARKS

The pace of experimental progress in this field is so rapid that some of the conclusions presented here could be obsolete by the publication date. Nevertheless, some conclusions have been established firmly enough to be summarized with some certainty. First, the physiological effects of opiates appear to be mediated by interactions with specific receptors located in synaptic membranes. The opiate receptors are part of one or more neuronal systems whose principal ligands are enkephalins and β-endorphin. The interactions of these peptides with receptors depend on strict conformational rules, although a precise map of the receptor active site will probably not be obtained without more information of the molecular nature of the receptor. A crucial question is what molecular events occur after binding of receptor and ligands; work by neurophysiologists to identify enkephalin actions on neurons as generally inhibitory in nature, as well as biochemical studies to identify opiate-inhibited adenylate cyclase, have begun to approach this question.

The relationship between enkephalin and β-endorphin is more complex than originally supposed. Despite their similarities in structure, the two peptides represent two different neuronal systems; indeed, β-endorphin may not even be a precursor of enkephalin. The functional significance of these separate pathways is not yet clear, and may be related to the question of multiple opiate receptors in the brain. It is clear, though, that enkephalin does fulfill many of the established criteria of neurotransmitters; enkephalinergic cells and fibers extend into a variety of brain areas, some of which mediate non-opiate-like effects. Some workers have preferred to call enkephalin a neuromodulator instead of neurotransmitter since the peptides appear to modulate the actions of other transmitters. Whether such distinctions are physiologically meaningful, or merely represent semantic differences, is a question that can only be answered by further research.

REFERENCES

Akil, H., Mayer, D.J. and Liebeskind, J.C. (1976), *Science,* **191**, 961–962.

Akil, H., Watson, S.J., Barchas, J.D. and Li, C.H. (1979), *Life Sci.,* **24**, 1659–1666.

Aono, J., Takahashi, M. and Koida, M. (1978), *Jap. J. Pharmac.,* **28**, 930–932.

Arbilla, S. and Langer, S.Z. (1978), *Nature,* **271**, 559–561.

Atweh, S.F., Murrin, L.C. and Kuhar, M.J. (1978), *Neuropharmac.* **17**, 65–71.

Audigier, Y., Malfroy-Camine, B.R. and Schwartz, J.C. (1977), *Eur. J. Pharmac.* **41**, 247–248.

Austen, B.M. and Smyth, D.G. (1977), *Biochem. biophys. Res. Commun.* **77**, 86–94.

Bajusz, S., Ronai, A.Z., Szekely, J., Graf, L., Dunai-Kovacs, Z. and Berzeti, L. (1977), *FEBS Letters,* **76**, 91–92.

Beddell, C.R., Clark, R.B., Hardy, G.W., Lowe, L.A., Ubatuba, F.B., Vane, J.R., Wilkinson, S., Chang, K.-J., Cuatrecasas, P. and Miller, R.J. (1977), *Proc. R. Soc. Lond. B.,* **198**, 249–265.

Belluzzi, J.D., Grant, N., Garsky, V., Sarantakes, D., Wise, C.D. and Stein, L. (1976), *Nature,* **260**, 625–626.

Bennett, J.P., Jr. (1978) *Neurotransmitter Receptor Binding.* (Yamamura, H.I., Enna, S.J. and Kuhar, M.J., eds), Raven Press, New York, pp. 57–90.

Bloom, F., Battenberg, E., Rossier, J., Ling, N. and Guillemin, R. (1978), *Proc. natn. Acad. Sci. USA,* **75**, 1591–1595.

Bloom, F., Segal, D., Ling, N. and Guillemin, R. (1976), *Science,* **194**, 630–632.

Blume, A.J. (1978a), *Life Sci.,* **23**, 759–762.

Blume, A.J. (1978b), *Proc. natn. Acad. Sci. USA,* **75**, 1713–1717.

Blume, A.J., Shorr, J., Finberg, J.P.M. and Spector, S. (1977), *Proc. natn. Acad. Sci. USA,* **74**, 4927–4931.

Bolme, P., Fuxe, K., Agnati, L.F., Bradley, R. and Smythies, J. (1978), *Eur. J. Pharmac.,* **48**, 319–324.

Bradley, P.B., Briggs, I., Gayton, R.J. and Lambert, L.A. (1976), *Nature,* **261**, 425–426.

Bradbury, A.F., Feldberg, W.F., Smyth, D.G. and Snell, C.R. (1976a), *Opiates and Endogenous Opioid Peptides.* (Kosterlitz, H.W., ed), North-Holland, Amsterdam, pp. 9–17.

Bradbury, A.F., Smyth, D.G. and Snell, C.R. (1976b), *CIBA Found. Symp.,* **41**, 61–75.

Bradbury, A.F., Smyth, D.G. and Snell, C.R. (1976c), *Biochem. biophys. Res. Commun.,* **69**, 950–956.

Buscher, H.H., Hill, R.C., Romer, D., Cardinaux, F., Closse, A., Hauser, D. and Pless, D., Jr. (1976), *Nature,* **261**, 423–424.

Caruso, T.P., Takemori, A.E., Larson, D.L. and Portoghese, P.S. (1979), *Science,* **204**, 316–318.

Chang, J.K., Fong, B.T.W., Pert, A. and Pert, C.B. (1976), *Life Sci.,* **18**, 1473–1482.

Chang, K.-J. and Cuatrecasas, P. (1979b), *J. biol. Chem.,* **254**, 2610–2618.

Cheung, A. and Goldstein, A. (1976), *Life Sci.,* **19**, 1005–1008.

Childers, S.R. and Snyder, S.H. (1978), *Life Sci.,* **23**, 759–762.

Childers, S.R. and Snyder, S.H. (1979), *CNS Effects of Hypothalamic Hormones and Other Peptides.* (Collu, R., Barbeau, A., Cicharme, J.R. and Rochefort, J.-C., eds), Raven Press, New York, pp. 253–260.

Childers, S.R. and Snyder, S.H. (1980), *J. Neurochem.,* **34**, 583–593.

Childers, S.R., Creese, I., Snowman, A.M. and Snyder, S.H. (1979), *Eur. J. Pharmac.,* **55**, 11–18.

Childers, S.R., Schwarcz, R., Coyle, J.T. and Snyder, S.H. (1978), *The Endorphins, Advances in Biochemistry Psychopharmacology,* Vol. 18; (Costa, E. and Trabucchi, M. eds), Raven Press New York, pp. 161–174.

Childers, S.R., Simantov, R. and Snyder, S.H. (1977), *Eur. J. Pharmac.,* **46**, 289–293.

Chretien, M., Benjannet, S., Dragon, N., Seida, H.N.G. and Lis, M., (1976) *Biochem. biophys. Res. Commun.,* **72**, 472–478.

Collier, H.O.J. and Roy, A.C. (1974), *Nature,* **248**, 24–27.

Cox, B.M., Goldstein, A. and Li, C.H. (1976), *Proc. natn. Acad. Si. USA,* **73**, 1821–1823.

Cox, B.M., Opheim, K.E., Teschemacher, H. and Goldstein, A. (1975), *Life Sci.,* **16**, 1777–1782.

Creese, I. and Snyder, S.H. (1975), *J. Pharmac. exp. Ther.,* **194**, 205–219.

Crine, P., Benjannet, S., Seidah, N.G., Lis, M. and Chretien, M. (1977), *Proc. natn. Acad. Sci. USA,* **74**, 4276–4280.

Crine, P., Gianoulakis, C., Seidah, N.G., Gossard, F., Pezalla, P.D., Lis, M. and Chretien, M. (1978), *Proc. natn. Acad. Sci. USA,* **75**, 4719–4723.

Cuello, A.C. and Paxinos, G. (1978), *Nature,* **271**, 178–180.

Cusan, L., Dupont, A., Kledzik, G.S., Labrie, F., Coy, D.H. and Schally, A.V. (1977), *Nature,* **268**, 544–547.

Davies, J. and Dray, A. (1976), *Nature,* **262**, 603–604.

DeWied, D., Kovacs, G.L., Bohus, B., Van Ree, J.M. and Greven, H.M. (1978), *Eur. J. Pharmac.,* **49**, 427–436.

DiGuilio, A.M., Yang, H.-Y.T., Lutold, B., Fratta, W., Hong, J. and Costa, E. (1979), *Neuropharmac.,* **17**, 989–992.

Duggan, A.W., Hall, J.G. and Headley, P.R. (1976), *Nature,* **264**, 456–458.

Duka, T., Hollt, V., Przewlocki, R., Wesche, D. (1978), *Biochem. biophys. Res. Commun.,* **85**, 1119–1127.

Dupont, A., Cusan, L., Labrie, F., Coy, D.H. and Li, C.H. (1977), *Biochem. biophys. Res. Commun.,* **75**, 76–82.

Dutta, A.S., Gormley, J.J., Hayward, C.F., Morley, J.S., Shaw, J.S., Stacey, G.J. and Turnbull, M.T. (1977), *Life Sci.,* **21**, 559–562.

Enero, M.A. (1977), *Eur. J. Pharmac.,* **45**, 349–356.

Fredrickson, R.C.A. (1977), *Life Sci.,* **21**, 23–41.

Fredrickson, R.C.A. and Norris, F.H. (1976), *Science,* **194**, 440–442.

Fredrickson, R.C.A., Nickander, R., Smithwick, E.L., Shuman, R. and Norris, F.H. (1976), *Opiates and Endogenous Opioid Peptides.* (Kosterlitz, H.W., ed), North-Holland Amsterdam, pp. 239–246.

Fry, J.P., Zielglgansberger, W. and Herz, A. (1979), *Brain Res.,* **163**, 295–305.

Gacel, G., Fournie-Zaluski, M.-C., Feelion, E., Roques, B.P., Senault, B., Lecomte, J.-M., Malfroy, B., Swerts, J.-P. and Schwartz, J.-C. (1979), *Life Sci.,* **24**, 725–732.

Gent, J.P. and Wolstencroft, J.H. (1976), *Nature,* **261**, 426–427.

Gintzler, A.R., Gershon, M.D. and Spector, S. (1978) *Science,* **199**, 447–448.

Gintzler, A.R., Levy, A. and Spector, S. (1976), *Proc. natn. Acad. Sci. USA,* **73**, 2132–2136.

Goldstein, A., Lowney, L.I. and Pal, B.K. (1971), *Proc. natn. Acad. Sci. USA,* **68**, 1742–1747.

Gorin, F.A., Balasubramanian, T.M., Barry, C.D. and Marshall, G.R. (1978), *J. Supramol. Structure,* **9**, 27–39.

Graf, L., Szekely, J.I., Ronai, A.Z., Dunai-Kovacs, Z., Bajusz, S. (1976), *Nature,* **263**, 240–241.

Greidanus, T.B., Thody, T.J., Verspaget, H., De Rotte, G.A., Goedemans, H.J.H., Croiset, G. and van Ree, J. (1979), *Life Sci.,* **24**, 579–588.

Gros, C., Malfroy, B., Swerts, J.P., Dray, F. and Schwartz, J.C. (1978), *Eur. J. Pharmac.,* **51**, 317–318.

Grube, D., Voight, K.H. and Weber, E. (1978), *Histochem.,* **59**, 75–79.

Guillemin, R., Ling, N. and Vargo, T. (1977a), *Biochem. biophys. Res. Commun.,* **77**, 361–366.

Guillemin, R., Vargo, T., Rossier, J., Minick, S., Ling, N., Rivier, C., Vale, W., and Bloom, F. (1977b), *Science,* **197**, 1367–1369.

Hambrook, J.M., Morgan, B.A., Rance, M.J. and Smith, C.F.C. (1976), *Nature,* **262**, 782–783.

Hazum, E., Chang, K.-J. and Cuatrecasas, P. (1979). *J. biol. Chem.,* **254**, 1765–1767.

Henderson, G. (1976), *Br. J. Pharmac.,* **57**, 551–557.

Henderson, G., Hughes, J. and Kosterlitz, H.W. (1978), *Nature*, **271**, 677–679.

Hill, R.G., Pepper, C.M. and Mitchell, J.F. (1976), *Nature*, **262**, 604–606.

Hokfelt, T., Elde, R., Johansson, O., Terenius, L. and Stein, L. (1977), *Neurosci. Letters*, **5**, 25–31.

Holaday, J.W., Dallman, M.F. and Loh, H.H. (1979), *Life Sci.*, **24**, 771–782.

Hong, J.S., Yang, H.-Y.T. and Costa, E. (1977). *Neuropharmac.*, **16**, 451–453.

Hosobuchi, Y., Rossier, J., Bloom, F.E. and Guillemin, R. (1979), *Science*, **203**, 279–281.

Houghten, R.A. and Li, C.H. (1978), *Int. J. Peptide Protein Res.*, **12**, 325–326.

Hughes, J.T. (1975), *Brain Res.*, **88**, 295–308.

Hughes, J., Smith, T.W., Kosterlitz, H.W., Fothergill, L., Morgan, B.A. and Morris, H.R. (1975), *Nature*, **258**, 577–579.

Huidobro-Toro, J.P. and Way, E.L. (1978), *Eur. J. Pharmac.*, **52**, 179–18\

Innis, R.B. and Snyder, S.H. (1979), *Ann. Rev. Biochem.*, **48**, 755–782.

Isogai, Y., Nemethy, G. and Scheraga, H.A. (1977), *Proc. natn. Acad. Sci. USA*, **74**, 414–418.

Iversen, L.L., Iversen, S.D., Bloom, F.E. Vargo, T. and Guillemin, R. (1978), *Nature*, **271**, 679–681.

Jacquet, Y.F. and Marks, N. (1976), *Science*, **194**, 632–635.

Jessell, T.M. and Iversen, L.L. (1977), *Nature*, **268**, 549–561.

Jones, C.R., Gibbons, W.A. and Garsky, V. (1976), *Nature*, **263**, 779–782.

Kangawa, K., Matsuo, H. and Igarishi, M. (1979), *Biochem. biophys. Res. Commun.*, **68**, 153–160.

Klee, W.A. and Niremberg, M. (1976), *Nature*, **263**, 609–611.

Knight, M. and Klee, W. (1978), *J. biol. Chem.*, **273**, 3843–3847.

Kosterlitz, H.W. and Waterfield, A.A. (1975), *Ann. Rev. Pharmacol. Toxicol.*, **15**, 29–47.

Krieger, D.T., Liotta, D. and Brownstein, J.J. (1977), *Proc. natn. Acad. Sci. USA*, **74**, 648–652.

LaBella, F., Queen, G., Senyshin, J., Lis, M. and Chretien, M. (1977), *Biochem. biophys. Res. Commun.*, **75**, 350–357.

Lad, P.M., Welton, A.F. and Rodbell, M. (1977), *J. biol. Chem.*, **252**, 5942–4946.

Lamotte, C., Pert, C.B. and Snyder, S.H. (1976), *Brain Res.*, **112**, 407–412.

Laubie, M., Schmitt, H., Vincent, H. and Remond, G. (1977), *Eur. J. Pharmac.*, **46**, 67–71.

Lazarus, L.H., Ling, N. and Guillemin, R. (1976), *Proc. natn. Acad. Sci. USA*, **73**, 2156–2159.

Lefkowitz, R.J. and Williams, L.T. (1977), *Proc. natn. Acad. Sci. USA*, **74**, 515–519.

Lemaire, S., Berube, A., Derome, G., Lemaire, I., Magnan, J., Regoli, D., and St-Pierre, S. (1978a), *J. med. Chem.*, **21**, 1232–1235.

Lemaire, I., Tseng, R. and Lemaire, S. (1978b), *Proc. natn. Acad. Sci. USA*, **75**, 6240–6242.

Lewis, R.V., Stein, S., Gerber, L.D., Rubinstein, M., and Udenfriend, S. (1978), *Proc. natn. Acad. Sci. USA*, **75**, 4021–4023.

Li, C.H. (1964), *Nature*, **201**, 924–925.

Li, C.H. and Chung, D. (1976), *Proc. natn. Acad. Sci. USA*, **73**, 1145–1148.

Li, C.H., Rao, A.J., Doneen, B.A. and Yamashiro, D. (1977), *Biochem. biophys. Res. Commun.,* **75**, 576–580.

Li, C.H., Tseng, L.-F. and Yamashiro, D. (1978a), *Biochem. biophys. Res. Commun.,* **85**, 795–800.

Li, C.H., Yamashiro, D., Tseng, L.F. and Loh, H.H. (1978b), *Int. J. peptide protein Res.,* **11**, 154–158.

Liotta, A.S., Gildersleeve, D., Brownstein, M.J. and Krieger, D.T. (1979), *Proc. natn. Acad. Sci. USA,* **76**, 1448–1452.

Loeber, J.G., Verhoef, J., Burbach, J.P.H. and Witter, A. (1979), *Biochem. biophys. Res. Commun.,* **86**, 1288–1295.

Loew, G.H. and Burt, S.K. (1978), *Proc. natn. Acad. Sci. USA,* **75**, 7–11.

Loh, H.H., Brase, D.A., Sampath-Khanna, S., Mar, J.B. and Way, E.L. (1976), *Nature,* **264**, 567–568.

Loh, H.H., Cho, T.M., Wu, Y.-C. and Way, E.L. (1974), *Life Sci.,* **14**, 2231–2245.

Loh, Y.P. (1979), *Proc. natn. Acad. Sci. USA,* **76**, 796–800.

Loh, Y.P. and Gainer, H. (1978), *FEBS Lett.,* **96**, 269–272.

Lord, J.A.H., Waterfield, A.A., Hughes, J. and Kosterlitz, H.W. (1977), *Nature,* **267**, 495–499.

Mains, R.E., Eipper, B.A. and Ling, N. (1977), *Proc. natn. Acad. Sci. USA,* **74**, 3014–3018.

Macdonald, R.L. and Nelson, P.G. (1978), *Science,* **199**, 1449–1450.

Malfroy, B., Swerts, J.P., Guyon, A., Roques, B.P. and Schwartz, J.C. (1978), *Nature,* **276**, 523–526.

Malfroy, B., Swerts, J.P., Llorens, C., and Schwartz, J.C. (1979), *Eur. J. Pharmac.,* **11**, 329–334.

Margules, D.L., Moisset, B., Lewis, M.J., Shibuya, H., Pert, C.B. (1978), *Science,* **202**, 988–991.

Marks, N., Kastin, A.J., Stern, F. and Coy, D.H. (1978), *Brain Res. Bull.,* **3**, 687–690.

Martin, W.R., Eades, C.G., Thompson, J.A., Huppler, R.E. and Gilbert, P.E. (1976), *J. Pharmacol. exp. Ther.,* **197**, 517–522.

Mayer, D. and Liebeskind, J. (1974), *Brain Res.,* **68**, 73–93.

Meek, J.L. and Bohan, T.P. (1978), *The Endorphins: Advances in Biochemistry and Psychopharmacology,* Vol. 18. (Costa, E. and Trabucchi, M. eds), Raven Press, New York, pp. 141–148.

Meites, J., Bruni, J.F., van Vugt, D.A. and Smith, A.F. (1979), *Life Sci.,* **24**, 1325–1336.

Miller, R.J., Chang, K.-J., Cooper, B. and Cuatrecasas, P. (1978a), *J. biol. Chem.,* **253**, 531–538.

Miller, R.J., Chang, K.-J., Cuatrecasas, P. and Leighton, J. (1978b), *Life Sci.,* **22**, 379–388.

Miller, R.J., Chang, K.-J., Cuatrecasas, P. and Wilkinson, S. (1977), *Biochem. biophys. Res. Commun.,* **74**, 1311–1318.

Miller, R.J. and Cuatrecasas, P. (1978), *Vitamins and Hormones,* **36**, 297–382.

Minneman, K.P. and Iversen, L.L. (1976), *Nature,* **262**, 313–314.

Morgan, B.A., Smith, C.F.C., Waterfield, A.A., Hughes, J. and Kosterlitz, H.W. (1976), *J. Pharm. Pharmac.,* **28**, 660–661.

Morin, O., Caron, M.G., DeLean, A. and LaBrie, F. (1976), *Biophys. Biochem. Res. Commun.*, **73**, 940–946.

Mudge, A.W., Leeman, S.E. and Fischbach, G.D. (1979), *Proc. natn. Acad. Sci. USA*, **76**, 526–530.

Mukherjee, C. and Lefkowitz, R.J. (1976), *Proc. natn. Acad. Sci. USA*, **73**, 1494–1498.

Nakanishi, S. (1978), *Proc. natn. Acad. Sci. USA*, **75**, 6021–6025.

Nakanishi, S., Inoue, A., Kita, T., Nakamura, M., Chang, A.C.Y., Cohen, S.N. and Numa, S. (1979), *Nature*, **278**, 423–427.

Nakanishi, S., Inoue, A., Taii, S. and Numa, S. (1977), *FEBS Letters*, **84**, 105–109.

Nicoll, R., Siggins, G. and Bloom, F. (1977), *Proc. natn. Acad. Sci. USA*, **74**, 2584–2588.

North, R.A. and Williams, J.T. (1976), *Nature*, **264**, 460–461.

Oka, T. and Sawa, A. (1979), *Br. J. Pharmac.*, **65**, 3–5.

Osborne, H., Hollt, V. and Herz, A. (1978). *Eur. J. Pharmac.*, **48**, 219–221.

Pasternak, G.W., Childers, S.R. and Snyder, S.H. (1980), *Science*, **208**, 514–516.

Pasternak, G.W. and Snyder, S.H. (1975a), *Mol. Pharmac.*, **11**, 474–478.

Pasternak, G.W. and Snyder, S.H. (1975b), *Nature*, **253**, 563–565.

Pasternak, G.W., Goodman, R. and Snyder, S.H. (1975c), *Life Sci.*, **16**, 1765–1769.

Pasternak, G.W., Simantov, R. and Snyder, S.H. (1976), *Mol. Pharmac.*, **11**, 735–744.

Pasternak, G.W., Wilson, H.A. and Snyder, S.H. (1975b), *Mol. Pharmac.*, **11**, 478–484.

Paton, W.D.M. (1957), *Br. J. Pharmacol. Ther.*, **12** 119–127.

Patthy, A., Graf, L., Kenessey, A., Szekely, J. and Bajusz, S. (1977), *Biochem. biophys. Res. Commun.*, **79**, 254–259.

Pedigo, N.W., Ling, N.C., Reisine, T.D. and Yamamura, H.I. (1979), *Life Sci.*, **24**, 1645–1650.

Pert, A. (1976), *Opiates and Endogenous Opioid Peptides*. (Kosterlitz, H., ed), North-Holland, Amsterdam, pp. 87–94.

Pert, C.B. and Snyder, S.H. (1973a), *Science*, **179**, 1011–1014.

Pert, C.B. and Snyder, S.H. (1973b), *Proc. natn. Acad. Sci. USA*, **70**, 2243–2247.

Pert, C.B. and Snyder, S.H. (1974), *Mol. Pharmac.*, **10**, 868–879.

Pert, C.B. and Snyder, S.H. (1976), *Biochem. Pharmacol.*, **25**, 847–853.

Pert, C.B., Bowie, D.L., Fong, B.T.W. and Change, J.K. (1976a), *Opiates and Endogenous Opioid Peptides*. (Kosterlitz, H., ed), North-Holland, Amsterdam, pp. 79–86.

Pert, C.B., Kuhar, M.J. and Snyder, S.H. (1976b), *Proc. natn. Acad. Sci. USA*, **73**, 3729–3733.

Pert, C.B., Pasternak, G.W. and Snyder, S.H. (1973), *Science*, **182**, 1359–1361.

Pickel, V.M., Joh, T.H., Reis, D.J., Leeman, S.E. and Miller, R.J. (1979), *Brain Res.*, **160**, 387–400.

Polak, J.M., Sullivan, S.N., Bloom, S.R., Facer, R. and Pearse, A.G.E. (1977), *The Lancet*, **ii**, 972–974.

Pollard, H., Llorens-Cortes, C. and Schwartz, J.C. (1977), *Nature*, **268**, 745–746.

Pomeranz, B., Cheng, R. and Law, P. (1977), *Exp. Neurol.*, **54**, 172–178.

Portoghese, P.S., Larson, D.L., Liang, J.B., Takemori, A.E., and Caruso, T. (1978), *J. med. Chem.*, **21**, 598–602.

Puig, M.M., Gascon, P., Craviso, G.L. and Musacchio, J.M. (1977), *Science,* **195**, 419–420.

Queen, G., Pinsky, C. and LaBella, F. (1976), *Biochem. biophys. Res. Commun.,* **72**, 1021–1027.

Reynods, D.V., (1969), *Science,* **164**, 444–445.

Roberts, J.L. and Herbert, E. (1977), *Proc. natn. Acad. Sci. USA,* **74**, 5300–5304.

Roemer, D. and Pless, J. (1979), *Life Sci.,* **24**, 621–624.

Roemer, D., Buescher, H.H., Hill, R.C., Pless, J., Bauer, W., Cardinaux, F., Closse, A., Hauser, D. and Huguenin, R. (1977), *Nature,* **268**, 547–549.

Roques, B.P., Garbay-Jaurequiberry, C., Oberlin, R., Anteunis, M., Lala, A.K. (1976), *Nature,* **270**, 618–620.

Rossier, J., Battenberg, E., Pittman, Q., Bayon, A., Koda, L., Miller, R., Guillemin, R. and Bloom, F. (1979), *Nature,* **277**, 653–655.

Rossier, J., French, E.D., Rivier, C., Ling, N., Guillemin, R., and Bloom, F. (1977a), *Nature,* **270**, 618–620.

Rossier, J., Vargo, T.M., Minick, S., Ling, N., Bloom, F.E. and Guillemin, R. (1977b), *Proc. natn. Acad. Sci, USA,* **74**, 5162–5165.

Rubinstein, M., Stein, S., Gerber, L.D. and Udenfriend, S. (1977), *Proc. natn. Acad. Sci. USA,* **74**, 3052–3055.

Rubinstein, M., Stein, S., Udenfriend, S. (1978), *Proc. natn. Acad. Sci. USA,* **75**, 669–671.

Schultzberg, M., Hokfelt, T., Lundberg, J.M., Terenius, L., Elfvin, L.-G. and Elde, R., (1978), *Acta Physiol. Scand.,* **103**, 475–477.

Schultzberg, M., Hokfelt, T., Terenius, L., Elfvin, L.-G., Lundberg, J.M., Brandt, J., Elde, R. and Goddstein, M. (1979), *Neuroscience,* **4**, 249–270.

Schulz, R., Wuster, M., Simantov, R., Snyder, S.H. and Herz, A. (1977), *Eur. J. Pharmac.,* **41**, 347–348.

Segal, D.S., Browne, R.G., Bloom, F., Ling, N. and Guillemin, R. (1977), *Science,* **198**, 411–414.

Shaar, C.J., Fredrickson, R.C.A., Dininger, N.B. and Jackson, L. (1977), *Life Sci.,* **21**, 853–860.

Shanker, G. and Sharma, R.K. (1979), *Biochem. biophys. Res. Commun.,* **86**, 1–5.

Sharma, S.K., Nirenberg, M. and Klee, W.A. (1975), *Proc. natn. Acad. Sci. USA,* **72**, 590–594.

Shaw, J.S. and Turnbull, M.J. (1978), *Eur. J. Pharmac.,* **49**, 313–317.

Simantov, R. and Snyder, S.H. (1976a), *Proc. natn. Acad. Sci. USA,* **73**, 2515–2519.

Simantov, R. and Snyder, S.H. (1976b), *Opiates and Endogenous Opioid Peptides.* (Kosterlitz, H., ed), North-Holland, Amsterdam, pp. 41–48.

Simantov, R. and Snyder, S.H. (1976c), *Mol. Pharmac.,* **12**, 987–998.

Simantov, R. and Snyder, S.H. (1977), *Brain Res.,* **124**, 178–184.

Simantov, R., Childers, S.R. and Snyder, S.H. (1977), *Brain Res.,* **135**, 358–367.

Simantov, R., Childers, S.R. and Snyder, S.H. (1978), *Eur. J. Pharmac.,* **47**, 319–331.

Simantov, R., Snowman, A.M. and Snyder, S.H. (1976a), *Mol. Pharmac.,* **12**, 977–986.

Simantov, R., Snowman, A.M. and Snyder, S.H. (1976b), *Brain Res.,* **107**, 650–657.

Simon, E.J. and Hiller, J.M. (1978), *Ann. Rev. Pharmac. Toxicol.,* **18**, 371–394.

Simon, E.J., Hiller, J.M. and Edelman, I. (1973), *Proc. natn. Acad. Sci. USA*, **70**, 1947–1949.

Simon, E.J., Hiller, J.M. and Edelman, I. (1975a), *Science*, **190**, 389–390.

Simon, E.J., Hiller, J.M., Groth, J., Edelman, I., (1975b), *J. Pharmac. exp. Ther.*, **192**, 531–537.

Smith, T.W., Hughes, J., Kosterlitz, H.W. and Sosa, R.P. (1976), *Opiates and Endogenous Opioid Peptides*. (Kosterlitz, H., ed), North-Holland, Amsterdam, pp. 57–62.

Smith, G.D. and Griffin, J.F. (1978), *Science*, **199**, 1214–1216.

Smyth, D.G., Massey, D.E., Zakarian, S. and Finnie, M.D.A. (1979), *Nature*, **279**, 252–253.

Snell, C.R., Jeffcoate, W., Lowry, P.J., Rees, L.H. and Smyth, D.G. (1977), *FEBS Letters*, **81**, 427–430.

Snyder, S.H. and Childers, S.R. (1979), *Ann. Rev. Neurosci.*, **2**, 35–64.

Snyder, S.H., Pasternak, G.W. and Pert, C.B. (1975), *Handbook of Psychopharmacology*, Vol. 5. (Iversen, L.L., Iversen, S.D. and Snyder, S.H., eds), Plenum Press, New York, pp. 329–360.

Sosa, R.P., McKnight, A.T., Hughes, J. and Kosterlitz, H.W. (1978), *FEBS Letters*, **84**, 195–198.

Spiehler, V., Fairhust, A.S. and Randall, L.O. (1978), *Mol. Pharmac.*, **14**, 587–595.

Suda, T., Liotta, A.S. and Krieger, D.T. (1978), *Science*, **202**, 221–223.

Swerts, J.P., Perdrisot, R., Malfroy, B., Schwartz, J.C. (1979), *Eur. J. Pharmac.*, **53**, 209–210.

Takahara, J., Kageyama, J., Yunoki, S., Yakuskiji, W., Yamauchi, J., Kagerjama, N. and Ofuj, T. (1978), *Life Sci.*, **22**, 2205–2208.

Taube, H.D., Borowski, E., Endo, T. and Starke, K. (1976), *Eur. J. Pharmac.*, **38**, 377–380.

Terenius, L. (1973), *Acta. pharmac. Tox.*, **33**, 377–384.

Terenius, L. (1978), *Ann. Rev. pharmac. Tox.*, **18**, 189–204.

Terenius, L. and Wahlstrom, A. (1974), *Acta Pharmac.*, *(Kbh.) (Suppl. 1)*, **33**, 55.

Terenius, L., Wahlstrom, A., Lindeberg, G., Karlsson, S. and Ragnarsson, U. (1976), *Biochem. biophys. Res. Commun.*, **71**, 175–179.

Traber, J., Fischer, K., Latzin, S. and Hamprecht, B. (1975), *Nature*, **253**, 120–122.

Tseng, L.F., Loh, H.H. and Li, C.H. (1976), *Nature*, **263**, 239–240.

Uhl, G.R., Childers, S.R. and Snyder, S.H. (1978a), *Frontiers in Neuroendocrinology*, Vol. 5 (Ganong, W.L. and Martini, L., eds), Raven Press, New York, pp. 289–328.

Uhl, G.R., Goodman, R.R., Kuhar, M.J. and Snyder, S.H. (1978b), *The Endorphins, Advances in Biochemistry and Psychopharmacology*, Vol. 18. (Costa, E. and Trabucchi, M. eds), Raven Press, New York, pp. 71–88.

Urca, G., Grenk, H., Liebeskind, J.C. and Taylor, A.N. (1977), *Science*, **197**, 83–86.

Van Ree, J.M., DeWied, D., Bradbury, A.F., Hulme, E.C., Smyth, D.G. and Snell, C.R. (1976), *Nature*, **264**, 792–794.

Van Ree, J.M., Smyth, D.G. and Colpaert, F.C. (1979), *Life Sci.*, **24**, 495–502.

Verhoeven, W.M.A., Van Praag, H.M., Van Ree, J.M. and DeWied, D. (1979), *Arch. Gen Psychiat.*, **36**, 294–298.

Viveros, O.H., Biliberto, E.J., Hazum, E. and Chang, K.-J. (1979), *Mol. Pharmac.*, **16**, 1101–1108.

Walker, J.M., Sandman, C.A., Berntson, G.G., McGivern, R.F., Coy, D.H. and Kastin, A.J. (1977), *Pharmac. Biochem. and Behav.*, **7**, 543–548.

Waterfield, A.A., Hughes, J. and Kosterlitz, H.W. (1976), *Nature,* **260**, 624–625.

Watson, S.J., Akil, H., Richard, C.W., Barchas, J.D. (1978), *Nature,* **275**, 226–228.

Watson, S.J., Barchas, J.D. and Li, C.H. (1977), *Proc. natn. Acad. Sci. USA,* **74**, 5155–5158.

Wei, E.T., Tseng, L.F., Loh, H.H. and Li, C.H. (1977), *Life Sci.,* **21**, 321–328.

Weissmann, B.A., Gershon, H., and Pert, C.B. (1976), *FEBS Lett.,* **70**, 245–248.

Weitzman, R.E., Fisher, D.A., Minick, S., Ling, N., Guillemin, R. (1977), *Endocrinology,* **101**, 1643–1646.

Yamashiro, D., Li, C.H., Tseng, L.-F., and Loh, H.H. (1978), *Int. J. Peptide Protein Res.,* **11**, 251–257.

Yang, H.-Y.T., Fratta, W., Hong, J.S., Digiulio, A.M. and Costa, E. (1978a), *Neuropharamc.,* **17**, 433–438.

Yang, H.-Y., Hong, J.S. and Costa, E. (1977), *Neuropharmac.,* **16**, 303–307.

Yang, H.-Y.T., Hong, J.S., Fratta, W. and Costa, E. (1978b), *The Endorphins, Advances in Biochemistry and Psychopharmacology,* Vol. 18 (Costa, E. and Trabucchi, M., eds), Raven Press, New York, 149–160.

Yeung, H.-Y., Yamashiro, D., Chang, W.-C., and Li, C.H. (1978), *Int. J. Peptide Protein Res.,* **12**, 42–46.

Zieglgansberger, W. and Bayerl, H. (1976), *Brain Res.,* **115**, 111–128.

Zieglgansberger, W. and Frey, J.P. (1976), *Opiates and Endogenous Opioid Peptides.* (Kosterlitz, H., ed), North-Holland, Amsterdam, pp. 231–238.

Zieglgansberger, W. and Tulloch, I.F. (1979), *Brain Res.,* **167**, 53–64.

5 Other Peptide Receptors

DAVID R. BURT

Abbreviations

AII	angiotensin II
SFO	subfornical organ
OVLT	organum vasculosum of the lamina terminalis
AP	area postrema
CSF	cerebrospinal fluid
B_{max}	concentration of binding sites
K_D	equilibrium dissociation constant
k_{-1}	rate constant for dissociation
k_1	rate constant for association
IC_{50}	concentration that inhibits binding by 50 per cent
SHR	spontaneously hypertensive rats
NT	neurotensin
BN	bombesin
VIP	vasoactive intestinal peptide
TRH	thyroliberin
CNS	central nervous system
SS	somatostatin

Acknowledgements

The author wishes to thank Dr Richard L. Taylor for review and comments on the manuscript and Ms Evelyn Rojas for assistance in its preparation. Portions of original research reported in this review were supported by U.S.P.H.S. grant MH-29671.

Neurotransmitter Receptors Part 1
(*Receptors and Recognition*, Series B, Volume 9)
Edited by S.J. Enna and H.I. Yamamura
Published in 1980 by Chapman and Hall, 11 New Fetter Lane,
London EC4P 4EE

5.1 INTRODUCTION

This chapter will critically review attempts to identify receptors for a miscellaneous group of small peptides with apparent multiple roles in the body, only one of which may be that of a neurotransmitter. Most appear to be present in the gut and thus belong to the group of brain-gut peptides (Pearse 1976, 1978). Peptides to be discussed in detail include angiotensin, neurotensin, bombesin, vasoactive intestinal peptide, thyroliberin, and somatostatin. Although evidence implicating them as neurotransmitter candidates is far from complete, all appear to be present in the central nervous sytem and to be localized to specific groups of neurons as judged by immunohistochemistry. It should be noted, however, that immunochemical techniques most commonly used to identify and measure these peptides do not preclude the possibility that in some cases a structurally related, perhaps larger, peptide is being measured in addition to or instead of the identified peptide. Identified receptors in brain thus may be responding in part or wholly to the related peptide *in vivo*.

The review will concentrate on demonstration of receptors by binding of radioactive peptides rather than by eliciting responses to applied peptides, although a response is, of course, necessary to attach any significance to binding. No attempt will be made to discuss mechanisms of responses, since information in this area is still almost totally lacking. Many related points will be referenced by other reviews.

The usual criteria for receptor identification by binding (Burt, 1978a; Cuatrecasas, 1976) include high affinity, appropriate kinetics, appropriate regional distribution and appropriate pharmacology. In the early stages of studying a brain peptide such as those in this chapter, what is 'appropriate' for its receptors may not be known. This is especially true of receptor pharmacology, since binding measurements are much easier to quantify than electrophysiological effects of iontophoretic application and easier to interpret than behavioral effects of local or systemic injection. Thus, in some cases, binding studies may give the first reliable information about the detailed pharmacology of brain receptors.

In the case of peptides well-characterized as hormones in peripheral systems, such as angiotensin II, thyroliberin, and somatostatin, it is potentially useful to compare the pharmacology and other characteristics of binding sites in brain with what is known of peripheral receptors. A close resemblance strongly suggests the brain binding sites are also receptors. Of course, a dissimilarity between brain binding sites and peripheral receptors does not necessarily mean the brain sites are not receptors.

5.2　ANGIOTENSIN

5.2.1　Background

Angiotensin is best known for its peripheral effects, particularly in relation
to hypertension, but has central actions as well (see Peach, 1977, for
review). Peripheral angiotensin derives from the well-known production of
renin by juxtaglomerular cells of the kidney (Fig. 5.1), which acts on
angiotensinogen, a protein from liver, in the circulation to yield the
decapeptide angiotensin I. The C-terminal His-Leu of angiotensin I is
removed by angiotensin-converting enzyme, predominantly in the lungs, to
yield the octapeptide angiotensin II (AII, Asp-Arg-Val-Tyr-Ile-His-Pro-Phe),
the major active species. Peripheral actions of angiotensins include
contraction of vascular and uterine smooth muscle, release of aldosterone
from adrenal cortex and release of catecholamines from adrenal medulla
and sympathetic endings.

　　Central actions of AII (Table 5.1) gave reason to expect the presence of
angiotensin receptors in brain long before they were demonstrated by
binding studies. Thus AII has central vasopressor actions and is a potent
dipsogen and releaser of vasopressin (see Severs and Daniels-Severs, 1973
for review of earlier studies). Possible additional central actions
of AII include effects on sympathetic activation (Hoffman *et al.*, 1977b), salt
appetite (Epstein, 1978) and secretion of corticotropin (Reid and Day,
1977). An important question is whether central receptors for AII are
binding only the circulating hormone or whether AII also is generated
locally in the brain as a possible neurotransmitter or neuromodulator,
justifying its inclusion in this chapter.

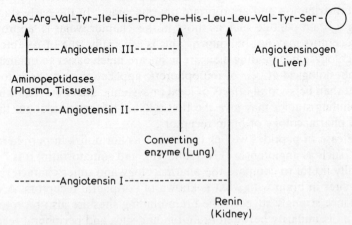

Fig. 5.1　The renin–angiotensin system.

Table 5.1 Central actions of angiotensin.

Stimulates thirst and drinking.

Increases release of vasopressin (ADH).

Raises blood pressure.

Activates sympathetic nervous system.

Increases appetite for salt.

Increases release of corticotropin (ACTH).

After some controversy (Reid, 1977), it has now been demonstrated to the satisfaction of most investigators that the brain contains a complete renin-angiotensin system (reviewed in Ganten and Speck, 1978; Phillips, 1978a). Immunohistochemical studies have found widely distributed neuronal cell bodies and terminals which react with antiserum against AII (Changaris *et al.*, 1978, Fuxe *et al.*, 1976, Nahmod *et al.*, 1977). Areas found to contain AII-like immunoreactivity in the central nervous system are listed in Table 5.2. Portions of the peripheral nervous system are also labeled. Overall levels of AII and possibly related peptides in the brain appear to be quite low, 0.7 pmol/g wet weight in the hypothalamus and 0.1 to 0.2 pmol/g in several other regions by radioreceptor assay (Snyder, 1978a, b). Yet there remains little doubt that many central angiotensin receptors, inaccessible to circulating AII, are responding to locally produced and released peptide.

The receptors which appear accessible to circulating AII in physiological

Table 5.2 Distribution of angiotensin II-like immunoreactivity in the central nervous system of the rat (adapted from Ganten *et al.*, 1978).

High density: Substantia gelatinosa of the spinal cord, nucleus tractus spinalis nervi trigemini, median eminence (medial external layer), nucleus amygdaloideus centralis, sympathetic lateral column.

Low–moderate density: Nucleus dorsomedialis hypothalami, locus coeruleus, ventral and caudal part of nucleus caudatus putamen.

Scattered terminals: Periventricular mesencephalic gray, hypothalamus, preoptic area, subcortical limbic structures (amygdaloid cortex, septal area), limbic cortex, thalamus (midline area), ventral midbrain, substantia nigra, reticular formation including the region of norepinephrine and epinephrine cell groups Al and Cl, respectively, in the ventrolateral reticular formation of medulla oblongata, raphe region, nucleus tractus solitarius, nucleus dorsalis motorius nervi vagi, periventricular area of pons and medulla oblongata.

No immunofluorescence: Parts of the neocortex, cortex cerebelli.

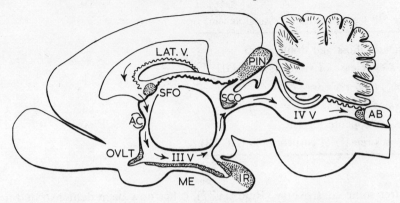

Fig. 5.2 Circumventricular organs of the rat brain. Abbreviations: AC, anterior commissure; OVLT, organum vasculosum of the lamina terminalis; ME, median eminence; III V, third ventricle; IR, infundibular recess and hypophysis; SCO, subcommisural organ; PIN, pineal gland; IV V, fourth ventricle; AP, area postrema; Lat V, lateral ventricle; SFO, subfornical organ. Arrows show direction of net flow of cerebrospinal fluid. (Redrawn from Phillips *et al.*, 1977a.)

doses are those functionally outside the blood–brain barrier in the circumventricular organs (Fig. 5.2), particularly the subfornical organ (SFO), organum vasculosum of the lamina terminalis (OVLT), subcommisural organ, and area postrema (AP). The SFO in the anterior third ventricle has been implicated in the dipsogenic effects of circulating AII (Simpson *et al.*, 1978), while the AP is implicated in its central vasopressor actions (Ferrario *et al.*, 1972). Receptors inaccessible to peripheral AII because of the blood–brain barrier seem to serve similar functions in many cases, but in some areas their functions are completely unknown.

This area of investigation has been confused because local injection of AII, if any leaks into the ventricles, can result in the injected AII gaining access to wide areas of the brain. Lesion experiments and experiments in which access of cerebrospinal fluid (CSF) to various areas of ventricular surface is prevented by cream plugs have suggested that the OVLT area is critical for both dipsogenic and pressor responses to AII in the ventricles (Phillips, 1978a). In addition, local injections have implicated the preoptic area, septal region, anterior hypothalamus and possibly other regions bordering the anterior third ventricle in angiotensin-induced thirst (Mogensen and Kucharczyk, 1978). Some workers have also suggested that central pressor effects of AII are mediated through receptors near the cerebral aqueduct (Buckley, 1977; Sirett *et al.*, 1979; see later discussion). Interestingly, intraventricular injection of AII seems to have little or no effect on the AP, presumably because this area is accessible only to circulating AII. Tight junctions between the ependymal cells apparently can constitute a 'CSF–brain barrier' to AII in the ventricles. Thus, on the basis of physiological experiments, central angiotensin receptors can be considered as belonging to one or more of three groups: (1) those that are accessible to circulating AII, (2) those that are accessible to ventricular AII, and (3) those that are accessible to locally released AII. The last group, presumably the largest, is the least well understood. Many of these receptors probably have nothing to do with fluid and electrolyte balance, drinking behavior, or pressor effects.

5.2.2 Binding studies

Several laboratories have studied binding of ^{125}I-angiotensin II to brain membrane preparations in an effort to characterize central angiotensin receptors (Table 5.3). These studies appear to have been looking in large part at 'peripherally inaccessible' (or presumably neurotransmission-related) receptors because the circumventricular organs represent so little tissue.

The initial report (Bennett and Snyder, 1976) dealt in greatest detail with calf cerebellar cortex, which proved to have the highest concentration of binding sites (B_{max}) for ^{125}I-AII of any bovine or rat tissue or brain region examined, about 1.6 pmol/g wet weight. Interestingly, the rat cerebellum proved to have many fewer sites. Indeed, binding in rat thalamus-hypothalamus, midbrain and brainstem was higher than rat cerebellum. So long as the functions of AII in the cerebellum, and thus the properties to be expected of its receptors there, are still completely unknown, no convincing proof of receptor identity is possible.

Demonstrated characteristics of binding were consistent with receptor identification. Several means of reducing peptidase activity were combined to permit incubations at 37° C without appreciable ligand degradation. Intactness of bound radioactivity was checked not only by thin layer chromatography but also by its ability to rebind to fresh membranes. Differential centrifugation of teflon-glass homogenates in 0.32 M sucrose localized 75 per cent of the recovered binding to the crude mitochondrial fraction, consistent with what has been found for most other neurotransmitter receptors. The routine tissue preparation, however, was a total particulate fraction. In the presence of Na^+ approaching physiological concentrations, only a single class of high affinity ^{125}I-AII binding sites, with an equilibrium dissociation constant (K_D) of about 0.2 nM by saturation analysis, was reported in calf cerebellar cortex membranes. A similar value was obtained by competition of unlabeled AII, suggesting that the iodination had little effect on the molecule's ability to bind. The measured rate constant for dissociation (k_{-1}), 1.6×10^{-2} min^{-1}, divided by the rate

Table 5.3 Binding studies of angiotensin receptors in brain.

Ligand	K_D	B_{max}	Region	Species	Temp. (°C)	k_1 (M^{-1} min^{-1})	k_{-1} (min^{-1})	Comments	Reference
^{125}I-AII	0.2 nM	1.6 pmol/gww	cerebellar cortex	bovine	37	1.8×10^8	0.016	Analogs show 10× greater absolute potencies than in adrenal cortex, relative potencies similar	Bennett and Snyder (1976)
			(thalamus-hypothalamus)	(rat)					
^{125}I-AII	0.08, 0.5 nM (150 nM Na$^+$)	1.2, 2.0 pmol/gww	cerebellar cortex	bovine	37	$8{-}16 \times 10^8$	0.02	Analog specificity closely resembles rabbit uterus, but uterus lacks Na$^+$ enhancement of binding	Bennett and Snyder (1980)
^{125}I-AII	0.4, 3 nM (10 mM Na$^+$)	0.3, 1.5 pmol/gww	cerebellar cortex	bovine	37	5×10^8	0.06, 0.02		
[125]I-[Sar^1 Leu^8]AII	0.03, 0.04 nM (150 mM Na$^+$)	0.4, 1.8 pmol/gww	cerebellar cortex	bovine	37	9.1×10^8	0.017	Very similar to use of ^{125}I-AII	
^{125}I-AII	0.9 nM	11 fmol / mg protein	hypothalamus-thalamus-septum-midbrain (HTSM)	rat	22	1.1×10^8	(>0.7)	Highest binding in lateral septal area, high in area postrema	Sirett et al. (1977)
^{125}I-AII	—	—	superior colliculus	rat	22	—	—	Binding in superior colliculus equally high	Sirett et al. (1979)
^{125}I-AII	0.5 nM	12 fmol mg protein	HTSM	rat	25	—	—	No change in SHR	Cole et al. (1978)
^{125}I-AII	—	(0.24 fmol/mg protein)	OVLT	rat	not in abstract	—	—	Binding in OVLT up 127% in SHR	Stamler et al. (1978)
		(1.2 fmol/mg protein)	SFO						
		(0.13 fmol/mg protein)	cortex						

constant for association (k_1), 1.8×10^8 M^{-1} min^{-1}, gave a K_D of 0.09 nM, in reasonable agreement with the equilibrium values for this kind of study. Thus the binding was saturable, of high affinity, and reversible. The dissociation of bound AII, with a half time of about 45 min at 37° C, was certainly very slow for conventional neurotransmission. Relatively slow on and off rates tend to be typical of binding of this class of peptide.

The most interesting part of the study was the comparison of bovine cerebellar cortex binding sites with those in rat brain and bovine adrenal cortex. Although other laboratories had previously studied the characteristics of adrenal cortex binding (reviewed in Devynck and Meyer, 1978), the authors prudently did side-by-side experiments to get a more valid comparison. All three tissues showed fairly similar relative potencies for several angiotensin analogs, including the antagonist [Sar^1-Leu^8]-AII, but the two brain preparations had about ten times greater absolute potencies than the adrenal preparation. The recent finding that adrenal cortex appears to contain specific receptors for the heptapeptide angiotensin III ([des-Asp^1]-AII) as well as receptors for AII (Devynck and Meyer, 1978) may make the adrenal a less-than-ideal peripheral tissue for comparison.

No effort will be made here to review the detailed pharmacology of angiotensin receptors. This subject has been reviewed in depth for peripheral receptors (Khosla *et al.*, 1974; Regoli *et al.*, 1974) and unique features of central receptors seem to be rather subtle (see below). Many aspects of structure–activity relationships at peripheral angiotensin receptors are summarized in Table 5.4.

A more recent binding study by the same group (Bennett and Snyder, 1980) has extended the comparison to rabbit uterus and has added the use of ^{125}I-[Sar^1 Leu^8]-AII as labeled ligand. Most of the properties of binding of the antagonist ligand resembled those of ^{125}I-AII (Table 5.3). However, binding of the ^{125}I-[Sar^{1}Leu^8]-AII was less sensitive to enhancement by sodium ion in both bovine cerebellar cortex and bovine adrenal cortex. This reduced sensitivity to sodium appeared to be due to the sarcosine substitution in particular, designed to reduce lability to aminopeptidases, rather than to the antagonist properties of the molecule, which are due to substitution of Leu for Phe at position 8. The three tissues calf cerebellar cortex, bovine adrenal cortex and rabbit uterus could be clearly distinguished by the way their binding of ^{125}I-AII at a concentration of 50 pM responded to Na$^+$: the enhancement in going from 10 mM Na$^+$ to 150 mM Na$^+$ was respectively 25-fold, 2.5-fold, and 1-fold (no enhancement). It is interesting that rabbit uterus, which appeared to resemble calf cerebellum fairly closely in terms of its specificity for competition by angiotensin analogs (Fig. 5.3), diverged most widely in response to sodium. Adrenal cortex differed from cerebellum both in its reduced response to sodium and in its absolute and relative affinities for many angiotensin analogs (not shown).

Table 5.4 Structural features of angiotensin II (adapted from Peach, 1979).

1. Asp The structural importance of the NH_2 terminus is related to susceptibility to aminopeptidase and to receptor kinetics. The duration of action and perhaps potency are related inversely to the rate of hydrolysis of a NH_2 terminally substituted analog by aminopeptidase.

2. Arg This residue is important for receptor affinity and may function simply to extend the peptide chain to a more optimum length. The positive charge of the guanidinium side-chain is not requisite for biologic activity.

3. Val The aliphatic side-chain of this residue is important. It is thought that hydrogen bonding through the side chain contributes to the conformation of the peptide.

4. Tyr The phenolic hydroxyl and the aromatic side-chain are essential for receptor affinity and probably contribute to the intrinsic activity of angiotensin.

5. Ile A β-aliphatic or alicyclic side-chain is required of the no. 5 residue to maintain biologic activity. Apparently Ile or Val exerts a rigid constraint on the peptide backbone which is important for activity.

6. His This residue is important for optimum receptor binding. The importance of the imidazole group appears to be related to its aromaticity, nucleophilicity, and potential for ionic interactions.

7. Pro The rigid constraint of the pyrrolidine ring is felt to contribute to a preferred conformation for high receptor affinity. This proline residue also protects angiotensin II from hydrolysis by converting enzyme.

8. Phe The COOH-terminal amino acid must have a free carboxyl group and an aromatic ring for high intrinsic activity. Removal of the eighth residue results in an inactive heptapeptide. The aromatic ring is the key to biologic activity since its replacement by various aliphatic side-chains results in analogs with good receptor affinity which essentially are devoid of activity on vascular smooth muscle.

Minimum peptide chain required for full biological activity = 3–8.

These more recent results also differed from the initial report in that saturation of high-affinity ^{125}I-AII binding to calf cerebellar cortex in the presence of 150 mM Na^+ was resolved into two distinct components, with apparent K_Ds of 0.08 and 0.46 nM and apparent B_{max}s of 1.2 and 2.0 pmol/g wet weight. The above values were read directly from the asymptotes of a curved Scatchard plot, with no correction for site–site interaction (Klotz and Hunston, 1971), so that the highest affinity site is presumably of even higher affinity than the 0.08 nM figure would indicate. With 0.05 nM ^{125}I-AII and 150 mM Na^+, only monophasic association and dissociation curves were obtained, with the ratio of the apparent rate constants, k_{-1}/k_1 (0.02 min^{-1}/1.1 × 10^9 M^{-1} min^{-1}), giving a value, 0.018 nM, somewhat lower

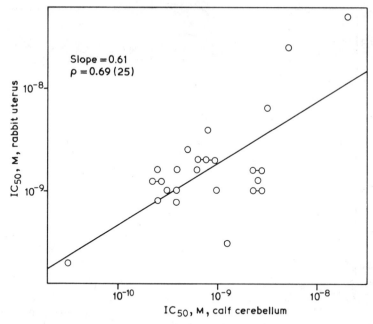

Fig. 5.3 Pharmacological comparison of ^{125}I-AII binding in calf cerebellum with that in rabbit uterus in the presence of 150 mM Na$^+$. Mean IC$_{50}$s of 25 analogs in each tissue are plotted against each other on a log–log scale. (Drawn from data tabulated in Bennett and Snyder, 1980.)

than the 0.08 nM high-affinity K_D read from the asymptote. These results would be nicely consistent with the presence of a very high-affinity site in cerebellum (K_D in 20 to 80 pM range) except that competition experiments were able to detect only the lower affinity site (K_D = 0.4 to 0.5 nM). The authors were unable to explain this anomaly. The effect of reducing sodium (Fig. 5.4), when analysed by Scatchard plots, was to make the apparent high-affinity (0.08 nM) site disappear, to reduce the number of 0.4 to 0.5 nM sites about 7-fold, and to expose new sites of still lower affinity (K_D = 3 nM, B_{max} = 1.5 pmol/gww). The physiological significance of these complex findings is not clear at present, but it is of possible relevance that the dipsogenic effect of Na$^+$ in the ventricles is greatly enhanced by low doses of AII (reviewed in Andersson, 1978), i.e. there is physiological as well as biochemical evidence for strong synergism between Na$^+$ and AII in the brain. The results of the detailed comparison of cerebellar cortex binding sites for angiotensin with those in other tissues do seem to indicate that brain binding sites, and thus, presumably, brain angiotensin receptors, are unique in at least some of their features.

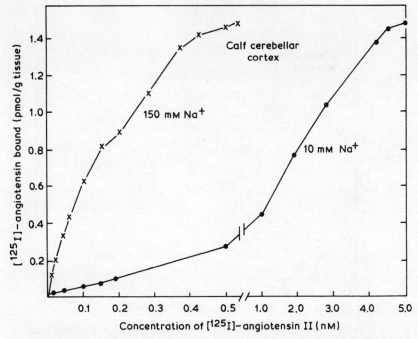

Fig. 5.4 Effect of sodium concentration on saturation of ^{125}I-AII binding to membranes of calf cerebellar cortex. (Redrawn from Bennett and Snyder, 1980.)

Other laboratories studying angiotensin receptors in brain have worked exclusively with rat brain and have concentrated more on trying to relate binding to known central effects of angiotensin than on detailed characterization of the binding itself. The initial report of this type (Sirett *et al.*, 1977) added the features of (1) a more detailed subcellular fractionation study, finding most binding in a crude microsomal fraction and relatively little in synaptosomes, (2) a more detailed study of regional distribution in rat brain, with highest binding in the lateral septal region, and (3) a demonstration of heat inactivation of the binding sites. This study found an apparent K_D of 0.9 nM for ^{125}I-AII binding to membranes of the hypothalamus-thalamus-septal-midbrains region of rat brain, with a B_{max} of 11 fmol/mg protein. In addition to the relatively small amount of binding associated with synaptosomal membranes, problems with the study include the facts that only two-thirds of the specific binding was reversible by adding nonradiactive AII, that this reversible binding was lost within 1 min at 22° C, and that total binding was lowered by about 25 per cent by 10^{-9}, 10^{-8}, or 10^{-7} M vasopressin and corticotropin. The reported rapid dissociation is desirable for a neurotransmitter candidate but is not

compatible with the reported high-affinity of binding and k_1 of
$1.1 \times 10^8 \, M^{-1} \, min^{-1}$ (22° C). No explanation for why the two unrelated
peptides should compete for any binding of ^{125}I-AII is apparent, but it is
possibly relevant that as much as 10 per cent of the ^{125}I-AII in the
incubation may have been broken down. The authors did not test whether
the competition by unrelated peptides was additive to that by 50 nM
[Asn^{1}Val^5]AII, their usual blank.

The most useful part of the study was the fairly detailed regional
distribution of binding. Besides the lateral septal area, regions high in
binding included midbrain, thalamus, hypothalamus and medulla.
Compared to these regions, binding to the cerebral cortex, hippocampus
and striatum was relatively low. Although fairly high levels of binding were
found in the medial septum, containing the subfornical organ, and area
postrema of the medulla, most of the binding could not be specifically
related to known physiological effects of angiotensin. An observation of
possible interest to endocrinologists was that the anterior pituitary had a
high level of apparent angiotensin receptors. This, in conjunction with the
finding of high levels of apparent angiotensin terminals in the median
eminence (Fuxe *et al.*, 1976), suggests a possible direct releasing hormone
function of angiotensin on the pituitary. The presence of angiotensin-
positive cell bodies in the anterior pituitary (Ganten *et al.*, 1978) may
complicate this interpretation, however.

A later study by the same group (Sirett *et al.*, 1979) sought primarily to
relate number of ^{125}I-AII binding sites in various regions to centrally
mediated pressor responses elicited by local injection of AII in parallel
experiments. The authors found binding in the caudal part of the superior
colliculi as high as that previously found in the lateral septum. They were
able to demonstrate that local application of AII to the surface of the
superior colliculus elicited a pressor response that could be abolished by
lesions including this region and the underlying dorsal periaqueductal gray
and that such lesions also abolished the pressor response to intraventricular
AII. Because of the possibility that critical fibers of passage were damaged
by the lesion and other difficulties, these results are only a preliminary step
towards correlating receptor localization with function. This preliminary
correlation of central pressor effects with binding in or near the superior
colliculus thus joins the same group's claimed previous preliminary
correlation of drinking with binding in the septal area and pressor effects of
circulating AII with binding in the area postrema.

Another group (Cole *et al.*, 1978) has tried to detect altered number or
affinity of presumed angiotensin receptors in spontaneously hypertensive
rats (SHR). This search arose out of reports that intraventricular saralasin
([Sar^{1}Ala^8]AII), the most commonly used angiotensin antagonist, lowers
blood pressure in nephrectomized SHR (SP strain) but not in control rats

(Phillips *et al.*, 1977b) and that intraventricular AII gives a greater pressor response in SHR (Hoffman *et al.*, 1977a). Binding methodology was similar to the two previously discussed papers, with similar results (Table 5.3). Perhaps because they assayed the combined hypothalamus-thalamus-septal-midbrain area rather than any discrete smaller regions, they were unable to detect any binding increase in spontaneously hypertensive rats compared to normotensive control rats.

Very recently, a third group has attacked the same problem (Phillips, 1978b; Stamler *et al.*, 1978), assaying the OVLT and SFO areas of the anterior surface of the third ventricle and the cerebral cortex. They were thus looking at the specific area (OVLT) most strongly implicated in the pressor effects of intraventricular AII, as well as another area (SFO) implicated in its dipsogenic effects. They found a more than two-fold increase in ^{125}I-AII binding in OVLT of SHR compared to control rats, but had too little tissue to determine if the binding increase was due to an increase in receptor number or affinity. There was little difference between SHR and control rats for the other two areas. This finding is perhaps the strongest evidence to date of the physiological relevance of ^{125}I-AII binding in brain.

5.2.3 Future directions

There remain several weaknesses in the attempted demonstration that brain binding of ^{125}I-AII represents receptors for centrally released AII or related peptides. These result largely from an absence of data. Demonstration of release and other criteria for identifying AII as a transmitter remain to be satisfied. A detailed comparison of the regional distribution of binding with distribution of endogenous angiotensin or its associated enzymes in the same species has not yet been attempted. Many difficulties have arisen in attempting to measure angiotensin levels by radioimmunoassay (discussed in Phillips, 1978a; Reid, 1977), and it is already clear that much converting enzyme activity is not associated with ^{125}I-AII binding. For instance, the highest levels of converting enzyme activity in calf brain are in the globus pallidus, with the cerebellar cortex well down on the list (Arregui *et al.*, 1977). Similarly, it has not yet been possible to correlate the extent of binding in various regions with the proportion of neurons responding to iontophoretic AII. Finally, although the detailed pharmacology of binding in calf cerebellum is known, and has been compared to that in other tissues (Bennett and Snyder, 1976, 1980), available data on the pharmacology of drinking behavior (Fitzsimons *et al.*, 1978; Swanson *et al.*, 1973; and others) and of neuronal response to iontophoretic application (Felix and Schlegel, 1978; Phillips and Felix, 1976), while fully consistent, are not sufficiently detailed for a definitive comparison. Perhaps the most useful result of the iontophoretic experiments has been the demonstration that saralasin slows the background firing rate of AII-sensitive neurons as well as inhibiting the effects of AII (Phillips and Felix, 1976). It is also of interest that AIII gave a significantly higher stimulation of firing rate of neurons in the SFO than AII (Felix and Schlegel, 1978), which parallels the observation that AIII is more potent than AII in competing for ^{125}I-AII binding in both rat and calf brain (Bennett and Snyder, 1976). The best opportunity for a definitive pharmacological comparison between binding and response may lie in doing both in a well-chosen neuronal tissue culture system (Sakai *et al.*, 1974).

Even if angiotensin binding in brain can be fully established to represent receptors, there will remain many questions about (1) how this binding is coupled to a cellular response, (2) the time course of this response relative to that of binding, (3) what other transmitter systems or mechanisms are involved in coupling this response to behavior, (4) regulation of receptors, (5) whether receptors are presynaptic, i.e. on nerve terminals as suggested for sympathetic endings (Starke *et al.*, 1977). Many of these questions can be answered by biochemical approaches, but others lie in the domain of the electrophysiologist or histochemist. Technical advances, such as photo-affinity labeling of brain receptors (Escher *et al.*, 1978) and possible purification of receptors and preparation of antibodies against them, should help with some questions. A preliminary attempt to answer the last question for central catecholaminergic neurons has already been made by injecting 6-hydroxydopamine intraventricularly and looking for a decrease in ^{125}I-AII binding (Snyder, 1978a). None was detected.

There exists a general lack of knowledge of the roles of central angiotensin. Much effort to date has been devoted to sorting out the effects of brain AII from those of circulating AII on drinking behavior and central pressor responses, but relatively little effort has yet been applied to following up leads from histochemical or biochemical experiments. Thus the possible role of AII in cerebellum, suggested by the high level of binding in the calf, remains unexplored. A possible role of AII as a sensory transmitter, suggested by the loss of apparent angiotensin terminals in the substantia gelatinosa upon sectioning the dorsal roots (Ganten *et al.*, 1978) appears similarly ripe for exploration. The finding of apparent angiotensin fibers descending into the intermediolateral cell column of the spinal cord, and of additional fibers and possible cell bodies in sympathetic ganglia (Ganten *et al.*, 1978), both suggest an amazingly widespread involvement of neuronal angiotensin in blood pressure control. Low levels of AII binding have been reported in the spinal cord (Sirett *et al.*, 1979), but no regional localization or other experiments to attempt to correlate binding with possible sensory or other function have been attempted. The list could go on and on.

5.3 NEUROTENSIN

5.3.1 Background

Neurotensin (NT,pGlu-Leu-Tyr-Glu-Asn-Lys-Pro-Arg-Arg-Pro-Tyr-Ile-Leu-OH) is a tridecapeptide isolated from bovine hypothalami by Carraway and Leeman (1973, 1975a) on the basis of its production of local vasodilatation and hypotension. Its activity was noted serendipitously during the purification of substance P. Additional activities of NT in the periphery include contraction of rat uterus and guinea-pig ileum, relaxation of rat duodenum, increased vascular permeability, transient cyanosis, increased secretion of corticotropin, follicle cell stimulating hormone and luteinizing hormone, hyperglycemia and pain sensation (Carraway and Leeman, 1975b). NT also inhibits gastric acid secretion (Andersson *et al.*, 1976), elevates plasma levels of glucagon and decreases those of insulin (Brown and Vale, 1976) and increases plasma levels of growth hormone and prolactin (Rivier *et al.*, 1977). The latter effect seems to be exerted at the hypothalamic rather than the pituitary level (Rivier *et al.*, 1977), as does NTs effect on luteinizing hormone and follicle stimulating hormone (Carraway and Leeman, 1976a).

These apparent effects on releasing hormone secretion are the first of several central effects of NT listed in Table 5.5. Other central effects (reviewed in Bissette *et al.*, 1978a) include production of hypothermia by intracisternal injection (Bissette *et al.*, 1976; Brown *et al.*, 1977a; Loosen *et al.*, 1978), an effect much more potently produced by bombesin; enhancement of the sedative (and other effects) of barbiturates (Nemeroff *et al.*, 1977), an effect shared with somatostatin but opposite that of thyroliberin; reduction of locomotor activity (Nemeroff *et al.*, 1977); reduction of response to noxious stimuli (Clineschmidt and McGuffin, 1977, Clineschmidt *et al.*, 1979), an enkephalin-like effect (but it is not blocked by naloxone); neuroleptic-like muscle relaxation (Osbahr *et al.*, 1979); enhancement of the turnover of dopamine, norepinephrine and serotonin in various brain regions (Garcia-Sevilla *et al.*, 1978); and enhancement of the

Table 5.5 Central effects on neurotensin.

Apparent effects on hypothalamic releasing factor secretion.

Hypothermia.

Enhancement of barbiturate effects.

Inhibition of noiciception.

Enhanced turnover of brain monoamines.

Enhanced turnover of brain acetylcholine.

---

turnover of acetylcholine in certain brain regions (Malthe-Sørensen *et al.*, 1978). All of these central effects except the first-listed are produced only by central administration, i.e. NT administered intravenously is ineffective.

Although NT was originally isolated from the hypothalamus, it has since been found that in the rat, at least, the gut contains 95 per cent of total body neurotensin (Carraway and Leeman, 1976b), largely in the ileal mucosa. There it has been localized to a discrete class of endocrine cell, the N cell (Polak *et al.*, 1977).

NT may be a hormone in the gut, but in the brain it fulfills many of the criteria to be expected of a neurotransmitter or neuromodulator. Thus it (1) displays marked regional differences in its brain distribution as measured by radioimmunoassay (Carraway and Leeman, 1976b; Kobayashi *et al.*, 1977; Uhl and Snyder, 1976, 1977), (2) appears localized to discrete nerve cell bodies and processes by immunohistochemistry (Uhl *et al.*, 1977b, 1979), (3) appears concentrated in synaptosomal subcellular fractions (Carraway and Leeman, 1976b; Uhl and Snyder, 1976), (4) is released by a calcium-dependent mechanism from potassium-depolarized brain slices *in vitro* (Iversen *et al.*, 1978), (5) selectively inhibits neurons in locus coeruleus (Young *et al.*, 1978) and excites neurons in spinal cord (Miletic and Randic, 1978), (6) is rapidly inactivated by brain enzymes (Dupont and Mérand, 1978), and (7) possesses apparent receptor binding sites in brain, as discussed in the next section.

5.3.2 Binding studies

Three papers reported binding assays for apparent NT receptors in brain within a few months of each other (Kitabgi *et al.*, 1977; Lazarus *et al.*, 1977a; Uhl *et al.*, 1977a); and within 2 years of NTs sequence determination. No others have followed. Since all three try to cover the same ground, with somewhat different results, they will be discussed by topic rather than in sequence. In the following discussion, each will be identified by its first author's name only.

(a) Methodology

Methodological variations in the three papers are summarized in Table 5.6. All three used rat brain and added 0.5 to 2 per cent bovine serum albumin to their incubation buffer and rinse solutions. Blank tubes contained 1 to 6 μM non-radioactive NT. Two of the three decided to run incubations on ice to reduce peptidase activity. One group (Uhl) estimated specific activity of their ^{125}I-NT from its binding properties under the assumption that iodination did not affect its affinity. Thus they were able to compare the concentration of ^{125}I-NT giving half-maximal saturation with the concentration of NT giving half-maximal competition in the presence of a .

Table 5.6 Methodological variations in published studies of neurotensin receptors in rat brain (listed alphabetically).

Ligand	Temperature (°C)	Buffer	Tissue preparation	Incubation period (min)	Separation	Reference
[3H]-NT	24	50 mM *tris* HCl, pH 7.5	Synaptic membranes	30	Millipore filter (EGWP)	Kitabgi *et al.* (1977)
[125I]-NT	0	25 mM tris-acetate, pH 7.0	Synaptic membranes	5	Glass fiber filter	Lazarus *et al.* (1977a)
[125I]-NT	4	20 mM *tris* HCl, pH 7.5	Washed particulate	30	Centrifugation	Uhl *et al.* (1977a)

relatively low concentration of ^{125}I-NT. The other two groups do not state how their ligand's specific activity was determined, although both were running NT bioassays as part of these or related studies. The two groups with longest incubations (Kitabgi, Uhl) demonstrated absence of significant NT breakdown during their incubations by several criteria. Two groups (Lazarus, Uhl) reported inhibition of binding by physiological concentrations of various ions.

(b) Saturability
As shown in Table 5.7, all three groups observed saturable binding with K_Ds reasonably in agreement with each other, especially considering the variations in methodology.

(c) Reversibility and kinetics
All three groups found binding to be readily reversible, although only two gave detailed kinetic data (Table 5.7). One of the greatest discrepancies among the three papers was the much more rapid association and dissociation stated by Lazarus compared to the more detailed data of the other two groups.

(d) Distribution
Distribution studies encompass both subcellular distribution and regional distribution. The only subcellular fractionation study was by Lazarus, where highest specific activity of binding was found for membranes from a lysed crude mitochondrial pellet sedimenting between 0.4 and 0.6 M sucrose on a discontinuous sucrose gradient. This fraction conventionally is viewed as enriched in microsomal elements and synaptic vesicles, not synaptic membranes (Whittaker *et al.*, 1964).

   Two of the papers (Lazarus, Uhl) contained regional distribution data for ^{125}I-NT binding to rat brain, with some surprising discrepancies, even considering the different dissections and tissue preparations. Both agreed that the thalamus, hypothalamus, midbrain, and cerebral cortex had greater binding than the medulla-pons and cerebellum, in general accord with NT's regional distribution in rat brain (Carraway and Leeman, 1976b; Kobayashi *et al.*, 1977). The most detailed regional distribution study of binding was performed on calf brain (Uhl). Selected results of this study are tabulated with comparable results of the same group on immunoreactive NT in the same calf brain regions (Uhl and Snyder, 1976) in Table 5.8. Note that the major difference is an excess of levels over binding in hypothalamic and basal ganglia regions or, for different normalization, a relative excess of binding over levels in cerebral cortical regions. There are many points of similarity in the two distributions. Moreover, it can be argued that binding would tend to reflect number of innervated cells and their size, whereas

Table 5.7 Results of published studies of neurotensin receptors in rat brain.

Equilibrium K_D (nM)	B_{max}	Region	k_1 (M^{-1} min^{-1})	k_{-1} (min^{-1})	$K_D = \dfrac{k_{-1}}{k_1}$ (nM)	Reference
2	$\dfrac{135 \text{ fmol}}{\text{mg protein}}$	Hypothalamus–thalamus–brain stem	5.4×10^7	0.048	0.9	Kitabgi et al. (1977)
8	$\dfrac{440 \text{ fmol}}{\text{mg protein}}$	Not stated ('brain')	not given*	$(0.7–3)^\dagger$	—	Lazarus et al. (1977a)
3	$\dfrac{3.1 \text{ pmol}}{\text{g wet weight}}$	Cerebral cortex	2.5×10^7	0.09	3.7	Uhl et al. (1977a)

* Authors merely stated equilibrium was reached by 5 min (others reported about 30 min).
† Calculated from stated half-life of binding of 15 to 60 sec under different conditions.

Table 5.8 Comparison of regional distribution of ^{125}I-neurotensin binding (Uhl *et al.*, 1977a) with that of radioimmunoassayable neurotensin (Uhl and Snyder, 1976) in calf brain. In both cases data are expressed as percentage of values for frontal pole of cerebral cortex (neurotensin level = 1.8 pmol/g wet weight, binding = 13 fmol/g wet weight).

Region	Neurotensin level	^{125}I-Neurotensin binding
Cerebral cortex		
Parahippocampal gyri	375	177–188*
Cingulate gyrus (mid)	213	125
Frontal pole	≡100	≡100
Occipital pole	141	126
Precentral gyrus	136	97
Hypothalamus		
Anterior	962	144
Medial	1063	165
Mammillary bodies	617	132
Thalamus		
Dorsomedial	137	249
Ventral	71	136
Anterior	240	112
Pulvinar	79	99
Basal ganglia		
Caudate	613	100
Globus pallidus	519	84
Limbic regions		
Hippocampus	166	88
Amygdala	108	98
Brainstem		
Pons	69	50–68*
Medulla-oblongata	90	28
Colliculi	152	86–88*
Others		
Cervical spinal cord	59	13
Cerebral white matter	41	27
Cerebellar cortex	<18	31

* Range of values in more discrete regions.

levels would tend to reflect density of terminals in a region and that the two are not necessarily related in every case (Burt, 1978a). For a peptide neurohormone, which could travel an appreciable distance before hitting its receptors, e.g. in the cerebrospinal fluid, even less relationship between levels and receptors might be expected. A better comparison might be binding versus proportion of cells responding to applied NT, when such data become available.

(e) Pharmacology

All three groups tested the pharmacological specificity of their binding for various NT analogs, with a few gross disagreements for overlapping analogs (Table 5.9). The tremendous variation in results for NT_{6-13} and NT_{8-13} exceeds that which one could easily ascribe to methodological variation, especially in view of the relative agreement of the three groups for the K_D of the binding (see above). The only reasonable explanation is in terms of the purity or identity of some of the nominally identified neurotensin analogs. The Kitabgi group synthesized their own, the Lazarus group presumably did the same, while the Uhl group obtained their analogs commercially. All three groups noted some discrepancies between potencies in competing for brain binding and potencies in producing various peripheral responses

Table 5.9 Available data on pharmacology of brain neurotensin in receptor binding and comparison with relative potencies in producing hypothermia (all data as per cent potency relative to NT).

Analog	Binding			Hypothermia
	Kitabgi et al. (1977)	Uhl et al. (1977a)	Lazarus et al. (1977a)	Brown et al. (1978b)
Neurotensin (NT_{1-13})	≡100*	≡100	≡100	≡100
NT_{2-13}	—	185	—	—
NT_{4-13}	560	137	—	—
NT_{6-13}	1200	64	—	—
NT_{8-13}	560	7.7	0.03	—
NT_{9-13}	1.4	0.4	0.01	—
NT_{1-12}	0.01	—	—	—
NT_{10-13}	0.001	—	—	—
NT_{1-10}	≤0.001	—	—	—
[D-Pro^7]NT	—	—	3	100
[D-Arg^8]NT	—	—	107	100
[D-Pro^{10}]NT	—	—	0.6	<1
NT-NH-Me	—	—	0.03	<1
[Phe^{11}]NT	—	—	0.6	100

* Tabulated data are read from their Fig. 6.

(hypotension, hyperglycemia, hyperglucagonemia, increased vascular permeability), but only the Lazarus group, with the fewest discrepancies, ran these experiments in parallel. A more interesting comparison would be between the binding potencies of the analogs and their behavioral potencies, e.g. in producing hypothermia (Brown *et al.*, 1978b; Loosen *et al.*, 1978). Since the binding experiments are so much at variance with each other, it is probably premature to attempt a detailed comparison, at least when binding and behavioral experiments are done in different laboratories. The fourth column of Table 5.9 represents hypothermia-producing effects of NT analogs observed by the Lazarus group (Brown *et al.*, 1978b). Clear discrepancies are evident between the high effectiveness of [D-Pro^7]NT and [Phe^{11}]NT in producing hypothermia and their reduced effectiveness in competing for binding (Lazarus). Similarly, the authors state that [D-Tyr^{11}]NT, which is about ten times as potent as NT in producing hypothermia (data not shown), has no increased binding affinity. Relative behavioral potencies of analogs may reflect other factors besides affinity for receptors, such as agonist–antagonist character (intrinsic activity) and lability to peptidases.

(f) Comparison with other tissues
Only two binding studies of possible peripheral NT receptors have appeared (Lazarus *et al.*, 1977b; Kitabgi and Freychet, 1979). The binding sites in rat mast cells (Lazarus *et al.*, 1977b) are clearly distinct from those in brain in their lower affinity (K_D = 154 nM). However, the binding sites in longitudinal smooth muscle of guinea-pig small intestine (Kitabgi and Freychet, 1979) appeared quite similar to those in brain in their high affinity (K_D about 4 nM) and their relative affinity for 2 NT analogs. Thus [D-Arg^8]NT had a K_i of about 2 nM in the intestine versus 5 nM in brain, while [D-Arg^9]NT had a K_i of about 300 nM in the intestine versus 400 nM in brain. Interestingly, the effectiveness of NT and its two analogs in interacting with intestinal ^{3}H-NT binding sites matched very closely their effectiveness in producing tetrodotoxin-resistant relaxation of the longitudinal smooth muscle. The authors also demonstrated a lack of effect of NT on cyclic AMP or cyclic GMP levels in the smooth muscle preparation.

5.3.3 Future directions

Clearly so much remains to be done with central receptors for NT that there is no point in discussing the possibilities at length. They include (1) resolution of previously discussed discrepancies among the three published studies about kinetics, distribution and pharmacology of central NT receptor binding sites, (2) detailed comparison of resolved relative binding potencies

of NT analogs with behavioral and iontophoretic potencies and an attempt
to explain discrepancies, (3) detailed comparison of apparent peripheral
receptors in smooth muscle or other tissue with apparent central receptors.
Many other considerations are similar to those already commented on for
angiotensin. However, physiological studies of receptors for NT, and of
receptors for the four peptides yet to be discussed, suffer one major
disadvantage compared to studies of receptors for angiotensin. This is the
absence of pharmacological antagonists comparable to saralasin. In some
cases use of a specific antibody could provide similar information.
Nonetheless, discovery of a specific antagonist for any of these peptides
would be a major advance.

5.4 BOMBESIN

5.4.1 Background

Bombesin (BN,pGlu-Gln-Arg-Leu-Gly-Asn-Gln-Trp-Ala-Val-Gly-His-Leu-
Met-NH$_2$) is a tetradecapeptide originally isolated from frog skin (Anastasi
et al., 1971), where it is one of a family of six or more related peptides
(Melchiorri, 1978). Amphibian skin has proved a rich source of many other
peptides (Bertaccini, 1976; Erspamer and Melchiorri, 1973), including
angiotensin-like peptides, the neurotensin-like peptide xenopsin, and
thyroliberin, discussed later, so that the fact that BN was first discovered in
frog skin may be taken as a historical accident. The availability of antiserum
against BN soon allowed the demonstration of BN-like activity in
mammalian tissues, including gastric mucosa (Erspamer and Melchiorri,
1975), lung (Wharton *et al.*, 1978) and finally brain (Brown *et al.*, 1978a, b;
Villarreal and Brown, 1978). In rat brain, it has a heterogeneous
distribution resembling that of neurotensin, in that it is highest in
hypothalamus and very low or non-detectable in cerebellum. In both the
lung and gut, BN-like immunoreactivity is present in endocrine cells
tentatively identified as P cells (Polak *et al.*, 1978; Wharton *et al.*, 1978).
Peripheral effects of BN include increased blood pressure, contraction of
gall bladder, altered gastrointestinal motility and myoelectrical activity,
reduced feeding behavior, and increased secretion of gastric acid, gastrin,
cholecystokinin, pancreatic amylase, insulin and glucagon (Brown and Vale,
1979; Erspamer and Melchiorri, 1975), and pituitary prolactin and growth
hormone (Rivier *et al.*, 1978).

Central effects of BN (reviewed in Brown and Vale, 1979) include
extremely potent lowering of body temperature in rats exposed to cold
(Brown *et al.*, 1977a, 1978b); potent raising of plasma glucose, perhaps by
raising adrenal catecholamine secretion, which in turn lowers pancreatic

Table 5.10 Central effects of bombesin.

Hypothermia

Hyperglycemia
    Elevated glucagon
    Decreased insulin
    Elevated catecholamines

Stereotyped scratching

Inhibition of immobilization/cold stress-induced gastric ulcerations

Analgesia

Apparent inhibition of thyroliberin secretion by hypothalamus (in response to cold)

---

insulin and raises glucagon secretion (Brown *et al.*, 1977b); and other effects listed in Table 5.10. Brown and Vale (1979) have speculated that many central and peripheral actions of BN (or related peptides) may be unified by considering it a satiety factor involved in 'the behavioral and biochemical regulation of nutrient homeostasis'. They make an analogy with insulin, but a better analogy in the present context would be with the central and peripheral roles of angiotensin in blood pressure regulation.

Before turning to discussion of apparent BN receptors, it should be mentioned that they are presumably not receptors for BN itself. BN-like immunoreactivity in ovine hypothalamus appears to represent a 32-amino acid BN-like peptide extended at the *N*-terminus but closely resembling BN in its last 11 amino acids (Villarreal and Brown, 1978). A smaller form is also present in gut and plasma extracts (Brown *et al.*, 1978a).

5.4.2 Binding studies

A single study of apparent receptors for BN-like peptide(s) in brain has appeared (Moody *et al.*, 1978). The ligand used was [^{125}I-Tyr^4]BN, which was incubated with a brain particulate fraction at 4° C for 24 min before filtration through Whatman GF/B glass fiber filters to separate bound radioactivity. Despite pre-soaking the filters in 1 per cent bovine serum albumin, filter binding of 3 per cent of added radioactivity kept the saturable binding to tissue from greatly exceeding the blanks. Physiological NaCl concentrations (>100 mM) greatly inhibited binding, as was the case for NT.

Kinetic experiments yielded an apparent k_1 of 1.1×10^8 M^{-1} min^{-1} and k_{-1} of 0.1 min^{-1}. The ratio k_{-1}/k_1 yielded a K_D of 0.9 nM versus an equilibrium value from a saturation curve of about 5 to 6 nM. The B_{max} was 80 fmol/mg protein or 3.8 pmol/g wet weight in whole brain minus pons-medulla.

Table 5.11 Comparison of regional distribution of [^{125}I-Tyr^4]bombesin binding (Moody *et al.*, 1978) with that of bombesin-like immunoreactivity (Brown *et al.*, 1978a).

Region	Specific [^{125}I-Tyr^4]BN binding (fmol/mg protein)	BN-like immunoactivity (pg/mg wet weight)
Hippocampus	15.0 ± 2.5	3.4 ± 0.2
Striatum	9.5 ± 3.0	—
Cortex	9.0 ± 2.0	4.2 ± 0.1
Hypothalamus	8.5 ± 3.0	11.7 ± 1.3
Thalamus	7.5 ± 2.0	5.6 ± 0.3*
Midbrain	4.0 ± 1.5	
Cerebellum	3.5 ± 1.0	<1
Medulla/pons	2.0 ± 0.5	5.3 ± 0.5

* Thalamus and midbrain combined.

The regional distribution of [^{125}I-Tyr^4]BN binding sites in this study is shown in Table 5.11 next to similar data on the distribution of levels of BN-like immunoreactivity from Brown *et al.* (1978a). Even this crude tabulation shows some discrepancies, with a relative excess of binding in hippocampus and a relative excess of levels in hypothalamus. As already discussed for neurotensin, these discrepancies are probably not significant from the point of view of receptor identification. The authors also stated that the subcellular distribution of binding was consistent with localization to membranes from nerve terminals (data not shown).

The authors commendably presented data on pharmacology of both binding and induction of hypothermia for BN and 12 analogs (Table 5.12). Discrepancies are fairly minor and are easily ascribable to non-receptor factors. The fact that two analogs are more potent than BN itself on binding (but not on hypothermia) is less of a problem than it might be if BN itself were thought to be the endogenous neurotransmitter or neuromodulator. Moreover, the BN-like frog skin decapeptide litorin, while much less potent than BN in inducing hypothermia, is almost equally potent in producing hyperglycemia (Brown *et al.*, 1977b). Its 50 per cent binding potency (Table 5.12) is thus almost directly between the two disparate behavioral potencies. Presumably other analogs' binding potencies might better match their potencies in different measures of central response. Overall, the authors make a good case that the [^{125}I-Tyr^4]BN binding sites may represent the receptors for the central effects of BN-like peptides.

A subsequent paper (Jensen *et al.*, 1978) reported properties of

Table 5.12 Pharmacology of bombesin and related peptides for inhibition of [^{125}I-Tyr^4]bombesin binding to brain membranes and for central induction of hypothermia (per cent potencies relative to bombesin, IC_{50} = 20 nM; data from Moody *et al.*, 1978).*

Peptide	Relative potency to:	
	inhibit binding	induce hypothermia
[Tyr^4]BN	500	95
[D-Ala^5]BN	133	100
[D-Ala^{11}]BN	100	100
Bombesin (BN)	≡100	≡100
[D-Asn^6]BN	50	10
Litorin	50	5
Ranatensin	33	20
[Ac-Gly^5]BN	20	100
BN-OH	3	<1
[Tyr^{12}]BN	2	1
[D-Trp^8]BN	<0.2	1
[D-Val^{10}]BN	<0.2	1
Des-Leu^{13}, Met^{14}-BN	<0.2	<1

* Relative potencies calculated from their tabulated IC_{50}s.

[^{125}I-Tyr^4]BN binding to dispersed acini of guinea-pig pancreas at 37° C. The concentrations for half-maximal inhibition of binding (IC_{50}) by [Tyr^4]BN, BN, and litorin were 2, 4 and 40 nM, respectively. These concentrations resemble those observed by Moody *et al.* (1978) in rat brain (4, 20 and 40 nM, respectively), but the number of analogs tested were too few, and the conditions of the binding assay were too different for any statement about whether the presumed receptors in the two tissues are the same or not.

5.4.3 Future directions

Many possible comments here would be similar to those made for other peptides. Some of the most interesting avenues for future exploration have to do with the extent to which effects of activating BN receptors depend on other neurotransmitters. It has already been shown that BN-induced hypothermia can be reversed by centrally administered thyroliberin and

naloxone (Brown *et al.*, 1977d, 1978b) and that both BN-induced
hypothermia and hyperglycemia can be reversed by centrally administered
somatostatin (Brown and Vale, 1979). A degree of specificity in these
interactions is suggested by the fact that neurotensin-induced hypothermia is
not blocked by naloxone (Loosen *et al.*, 1978). Thus some of these
observations may offer clues to the types of neurons which contain receptors
for BN-like peptides.

5.5 VASOACTIVE INTESTINAL PEPTIDE

5.5.1 Background

Vasoactive intestinal peptide (VIP, His-Ser-Asp-Ala-Val-Phe-Thr-Asp-Asn-
Tyr-Thr-Arg-Leu-Arg-Lys-Gln-Met-Ala-Val-Lys-Lys-Tyr-Leu-Asn-Ser-Ile-
Leu-Asn-NH$_2$) is a 28 amino acid peptide isolated from hog duodenum
(Said and Mutt, 1970, 1972) and related in structure to secretin, glucagon
and gastric inhibitory polypeptide. Starting with the potent vasodilator and
hypotensive effects which gave it its name, the molecule has a wide variety
of biological actions in the periphery (reviewed in Said, 1975, 1978),
including (1) in the lung, relaxation of trachea and reduction of effect of
bronchoconstrictor agents; (2) in the stomach, inhibition of histamine and
pentagastrin-stimulated acid secretion, inhibition of pepsin secretion, and
relaxation of gastric muscle; (3) in the pancreas, stimulation of electrolyte
and water secretion and insulin glucagon and somatostatin secretion; (4) in
the liver, stimulation of adenylate cyclase and bile flow; (5) in the small
intestine, stimulation of secretion, increase in mucosal levels of cyclic AMP,
and smooth muscle contraction; (6) in the colon, stimulation of adenylate
cyclase and secretion. Peripheral distribution of VIP-like immunoactivity
includes the entire gastrointestinal tract from esophagus to rectum, and it is
also found in pancreas, adrenal gland, lung, placenta, mast cells and platelets.
In the pancreas and gastrointestinal mucosa it is partially localized to D$_1$
type endocrine cells (Buffa *et al.*, 1977; Polak *et al.*, 1974) but in addition is
widely distributed in the peripheral autonomic nervous system, particularly
in the superior and inferior mesenteric ganglia (Hökfelt *et al.*, 1977b), the
submucous and myenteric plexuses of the intestinal wall (Bryant *et al.*, 1976;
Larsson *et al.*, 1976b; Fuxe *et al.*, 1977b), nerves in male and female genital
organs (Larsson *et al.*, 1977) and nerves around cranial blood vessels
(Larsson *et al.*, 1976a).

   VIP-like immunoreactivity is also widely distributed in non-vascular
elements of the central nervous system (Besson *et al.*, 1979; Bryant *et al.*,
1976; Larsson *et al.*, 1976b; Said and Rosenberg, 1976), where it has been
localized to neurons and nerve terminals by immunofluorescence (Fuxe *et
al.*, 1977b). Subcellular fractionation studies also have localized VIP-like

Table 5.13 Central effects of vasoactive intestinal peptide.

Shivering.

Hyperthermia.

Hypotension.

Arousal effect on sleep electroencephalogram.

Altered release of hypothalamic releasing factors.

---

activity to nerve terminal fractions (Emson *et al.*, 1978; Giachetti *et al.*, 1977). Immunohistochemistry (Larsson, 1977) and subcellular fractionation (Emson *et al.*, 1978) both indicate a vesicular localization within the nerve terminal. Potassium-stimulated, calcium-dependent release of VIP has been demonstrated both in cortical synaptosomes (Giachetti *et al.*, 1977) and hypothalamic slices (Emson *et al.*, 1978). Iontophoretically applied VIP excites cortical neurons (Phillis *et al.*, 1978). Bath-applied VIP stimulates adenylate cyclase activity in membrane preparations of selected brain regions (Borghi *et al.*, 1979; Deschodt-Lanckman *et al.*, 1977) as it does in many other tissues. Other effects of centrally applied VIP (Table 5.13) include shivering and hyperthermia (Clark *et al.*, 1978), transient hypotension (Vijayan *et al*, 1979), an arousal effect on the sleep electroencephalogram (Said, 1978) and increased release of prolactin, growth hormone and luteinizing hormone mediated at the hypothalamic level (Kato *et al.*, 1978; Vijayan *et al.*, 1979). The last observation has been amplified by the recent demonstration that VIP inhibits K^+-stimulated release of somatostatin from hypothalamic slices (Epelbaum *et al.*, 1979) but is complicated by the demonstration that VIP itself is released into hypophyseal portal blood (Said and Porter, 1979). These items of evidence, as well as the binding studies considered in the next section, strongly suggest VIP as another peptide neurotransmitter or neuromodulator candidate.

5.5.2 Binding studies

Two laboratories have reported studies of apparent VIP receptors in brain (Robberecht *et al.*, 1978; Taylor and Pert, 1979), with considerably differing results (Table 5.14). The papers overlapped enough in what they tried to accomplish that they will be discussed by topic rather than in sequence.

(a) Methodology

Both groups used ^{125}I-VIP prepared by the chloramine T method from the natural peptide. Neither gave any data to establish the purity of the starting VIP or ^{125}I-VIP; neither demonstrated the intactness of bound or medium radioactivity after the incubations at 37° C for 10 (Robberecht *et al.*, 1978)

Table 5.14 Binding studies of VIP receptors in brain using ^{125}I-VIP.

K_D (nM)	B_{max}	Species	k_{-1} (M^{-1} min^{-1})	k_{-1} (min^{-1})	Reference
36	4 pmol mg prot.	Guinea pig	not calculated	not first order	Robberecht *et al.* (1978)
285	20 pmol mg prot.				
1	2.2 pmol g ww	Rat	1.3×10^8	0.12	Taylor and Pert (1979)

or 20 (Taylor and Pert, 1979) min. Both were probably deterred from these controls to some extent by the limited amounts of natural VIP available.

Robberecht *et al.* (1978) used pooled hypothalamus-thalamus-cerebral cortex from female guinea-pigs as the source of brain membranes while Taylor and Pert (1979) used male rat brains minus medulla, pons, cerebellum and midbrain. The guinea-pig membranes were collected at the 1.0 to 1.2 M sucrose interface from a density gradient centrifugation of an osmotically lysed crude mitochondrial pellet. The rat membranes were a form of total particulate. Only Taylor and Pert (1979) demonstrated linearity of binding with tissue. Aside from the species difference, the major methodological difference which might account in part for the differing results of the two studies was in the means of separating bound from free radioactivity: Robberecht *et al.* (1978) used relatively rapid (<20 s) filtration through Millipore filters while the other group used a relatively slow (>2 min) centrifugation through 0.32 M sucrose followed by a rinse centrifugation. The latter procedure would be unable to detect rapidly dissociating, lower affinity sites.

(b) Saturability
The major difference between the two studies was the 36-fold higher apparent affinity, K_D = 1 nM, Taylor and Pert (1979) found in rat brain from a saturation curve than Robberecht *et al.* (1978) found from a competition curve for the higher affinity of two observed sites in guinea-pig brain. Taylor and Pert (1979) observed an IC_{50} of 4 nM in competition experiments and saw no evidence for a lower affinity, saturable ^{125}I-VIP binding site.

(c) Reversibility and kinetics
In both laboratories, binding reached apparent equilibrium by about 10 to 15 min at 37° C, but only Taylor and Pert (1979) calculated a rate constant for association (Table 5.14). Another major difference between the two

studies was in the characteristics of dissociation of binding. Taylor and Pert (1979) observed a simple first-order dissociation reaction by addition of 0.1 μM nonradioactive VIP, with a half-time of about 7 min at 37° C. By washing and resuspending labeled membranes, Robberecht et al., (1978) observed a complex dissociation of at least two phases, with the faster phase resembling that seen by the other group. The second phase was so slow that 40 per cent of the initial bound radioactivity was still present after 1 h at 37° C. It is possible that at least a portion of the very slowly dissociating radioactivity may have been metabolized.

The on and off rates measured by Taylor and Pert (1979), with the on reaction largely complete in a few minutes and the off reaction having a half-time of 7 min, are not too inconsistent with the observations of Phillis *et al.* (1978) on the time course of excitation of cortical neurons by iontophoretic VIP. In the latter experiments, excitation sometimes took over a minute to develop and often lasted over a minute after cessation of application.

(d) Distribution

Taylor and Pert (1979) stated that their binding was enriched in synaptosome-containing subcellular fractions, while Robberecht et al. (1978) merely used synaptic membranes because that was what they had used in their previous work with VIP-stimulated adenylate cyclase (DeSchodt-Lanckman et al., 1977).

Only Taylor and Pert (1979) reported the regional distribution of binding. Their results are shown in Table 5.15 along with the recently reported regional distribution of extent of responsiveness of rat brain adenylate cyclase to 5 μM VIP (Borghi et al., 1979) and the most recently reported regional distribution of VIP-like immunoreactivity in rat (Besson et al., 1979). Table 5.15 shows several discrepancies among the three columns. Binding, cyclase stimulation and VIP levels are all fairly high in hippocampus and cerebral cortex, but there is clearly lower cyclase stimulation (on a per cent basis) in the striatum and higher stimulation in the cerebellum than would be predicted on the basis of the other two measures. The low proportional cyclase stimulation in the striatum is presumably due to the very high basal activity there, but the high stimulation in the cerebellum is unaccounted for. There is also lower binding in the hypothalamus than would be predicted on the basis of the other two measures. Less relative binding in hypothalamus than would be predicted by levels has been found for several neuropeptides and would be expected for those with possible releasing hormone function (Said and Porter, 1979).

(e) Pharmacology

The results of the only paper to test a number of VIP analogs (Taylor and Pert, 1979) are shown in Table 5.16. Robberecht et al. (1978) also found

Table 5.15 Comparison of regional distribution in rat brain of binding of ^{125}I-VIP (Taylor and Pert, 1979) with extent of VIP stimulation of adenylate cyclase (Borghi *et al.*, 1979) and with VIP-like immunoreactivity (Besson *et al.*, 1979).

Region	^{125}I-VIP binding (fmol/mg protein)	VIP stimulation of adenylate cyclase		Immunoreactive VIP (pg/mg ww)
		Difference*	%	
Striatum	10.0 ± 1.2	35	5 (ns)†	58
Hippocampus	8.6 ± 1.6	18	72	69
Cortex	7.5 ± 0.8	36	39	169–302‡
Thalamus	6.7 ± 1.0	—	—	34
Midbrain	3.2 ± 0.6	(3)§	(7)§ (ns)†	(24)§
Hypothalamus	1.1 ± 0.6	21	25	20–60‡
Cerebellum	<0.7	28–40†	43–88‡	nd.
Medulla/pons	<0.7	(3)§	(7)§ (ns)§	(24)§

* Units = pmol cAMP/mg prot. min.
† ns = not significant.
‡ Range of values in more discrete areas.
§ Midbrain and medulla-pons were assayed together as 'brainstem'.

Table 5.16 Pharmacology of binding of ^{125}I-vasoactive intestinal peptide (Taylor and Pert, 1979).

Peptide	IC_{50} to compete for ^{125}I-VIP binding
VIP	4 nM
Secretin	600 nM
[Gln^9, Asn^{15}]secretin$_{5-27}$	25 μM
VIP$_{10-28}$	45 μM
Secretin$_{5-27}$	200 μM
Secretin$_{14-27}$	300 μM
Secretin$_{15-27}$	800 μM
VIP$_{1-10}$, VIP$_{18-28}$, secretin$_{1-6}$	$\geqslant$50 μM

secretin to be 100- to 200-fold less potent than VIP, although their absolute potencies for VIP and secretin were about 10-fold less (IC_{50}s greater). There are unfortunately, as yet, no similar pharmacological data on relative potencies for stimulation of cyclic AMP formation in brain or behavioral or other central responses with which the binding data can be usefully compared. Both papers found VIP to be considerably more potent in inhibiting binding of ^{125}I-VIP than would be suggested by either published study of VIP's stimulation of adenylate cyclase (Borghi *et al.*, 1979; Deschodt-Lanckman *et al.*, 1977) or by its 10^{-6} M threshold in depolarizing dorsal roots and motoneurons in toad spinal cord (Phillis *et al.*, 1978).

Both groups also examined the effects of ions, with sometimes contrasting results. Robberecht *et al.* (1978) also studied the inhibition of binding by nucleotides.

(f) Comparison with other tissues

Extensive binding studies with ^{125}I-VIP in membranes and intact cells from liver, adipose tissue, intestinal epithelium and pancreas have recently been reviewed by Gardner (1979) and will not be considered here except to note a general similarity to the results of Taylor and Pert (1979). Several of the studies demonstrated a good pharmacological correlation of binding with stimulation of cyclic AMP formation in the same tissue. Apparent K_Ds reported in these papers ranged from 0.2 to 1.5 nM, much closer to the results of Taylor and Pert (1979) than those of Robberecht *et al.* (1978). In the absence of side-by-side experiments, it is not possible to state at present whether the receptor binding sites for VIP in any of these tissues are similar to those found in brain.

5.5.3 Future directions

The recent observation that VIP can lower blood pressure centrally as well as peripherally (Vijayan *et al.*, 1979) forms an interesting parallel with the opposite effect of angiotensin. Further pursuit of this parallel in terms of sites and mechanisms of the receptors involved in VIP's central hypotensive effects could prove rewarding. VIP's wide distribution in the sympathetic nervous system also presents something of a parallel with angiotensin and suggests many future avenues of experimentation as well as many possible future difficulties in sorting out receptors for its actions as a hormone from those for its actions as a neurotransmitter. Other comments are similar to those for peptides already discussed.

5.6 THYROLIBERIN

5.6.1 Background

Thyroliberin (thyrotropin releasing hormone, TRH, pGlu-His-Pro-NH$_2$) is a tripeptide isolated from the hypothalamus (Burgus *et al.*, 1970; Nair *et al.*, 1970) on the basis of its ability to stimulate release of thyrotropin (TSH) from the anterior pituitary. It was thus the first of the identified hypothalamic releasing hormones (Guillemin, 1978a; Schally, 1978). In contrast to the other peptides discussed in this chapter, TRH cannot be said to have a wide variety of effects in the periphery. Indeed, aside from its stimulation of prolactin as well as thyrotropin release from the pituitary (Tashjian *et al.*, 1971), only some fairly minor effects on gastrointestinal motility (Almquist, 1972; Morley *et al.*, 1979b), pancreatic endocrine secretion (Morley *et al.*, 1979a) and gastric acid secretion (Morley *et al.*, 1979b) have been reported in mammals. TRH-like immunoreactivity is present in the gastrointestinal tract and pancreas (Martino *et al.*, 1978; Morley *et al.*, 1977).

In the brain, TRH-like immunoreactivity was soon found to extend well beyond the hypothalamus (Hökfelt *et al.*, 1975; Jackson and Reichlin, 1974; Oliver *et al.*, 1974; Winokur and Utiger, 1974). Indeed 70 per cent or more of TRH in rat brain appears to be extrahypothalamic. All of this TRH appears to originate outside the hypothalamus, i.e. not be transported there in axons of hypothalamic neurons, in that extrahypothalamic TRH levels are unaffected by surgical isolation of the medial basal hypothalamus (Brownstein *et al.*, 1975b). The operation did result in a 76 per cent fall in hypothalamic TRH levels. Although most investigators agree that extrahypothalamic brain contains material which behaves like TRH in radioimmunoassays, bioassays, radioreceptor assays and some chromatographic systems (discussed in Jackson and Reichlin, 1979), it should be mentioned that there is still considerable controversy about whether most of this material is identical to the tripeptide TRH (Youngblood *et al.*, 1978, 1979). The situation is thus similar to that for several of the larger peptides in this chapter.

There is some evidence that the hormonal role of TRH may represent a relatively late evolutionary specialization, in that levels of TRH in amphibian blood, brain and skin are much higher than in mammals, but the pituitary–thyroid axis of amphibians and lower vertebrates is unresponsive to the molecule (reviewed in Jackson, 1978). Immunoreactive TRH is even present in circumesophageal ganglia of snails, which lack a pituitary (Grimm-Jørgensen *et al.*, 1975).

The wide distribution of TRH-like activity in the central nervous system and the tripeptide's apparent lack of thyroid effects in lower vertebrates are only two of many items of evidence suggesting an important role for TRH in brain function, possibly that of a neurotransmitter. Extensive studies of the central effects of TRH have been repeatedly reviewed elsewhere (most recently in Collu and Taché, 1979; Horita *et al.*, 1979; Prange *et al.*, 1979; Rastogi, 1979; earlier in Prange *et al.*, 1978a, b, c and many others), so that no real attempt will be made to do so here. Many effects are listed in Table 5.17, taken from Guillemin (1978b) and based on citations in Vale *et al.* (1977). Many of its behavioral effects seem to involve amphetamine-like activation. Recently reported additional effects of TRH include its antagonism of hypothermia induced by NT (Nemeroff *et al.*, 1978) and BN (Brown *et al.*, 1977d, 1978b) and its arousal of hibernating ground squirrels (Stanton *et al.*, 1978). Further pieces of evidence consistent with a possible neurotransmitter role for TRH include (1) its biosynthesis in brain (reviewed in Jackson and Reichlin, 1979; McKelvy and Epelbaum, 1978), (2) its synaptosomal localization (reviewed in Barnea *et al.*, 1977; McKelvy and Epelbaum, 1978; Terry and Martin, 1978), (3) its release by depolarizing stimuli (reviewed in Porter *et al.*, 1977; Terry and Martin, 1978), (4) its effects on neuronal firing rates (reviewed in Renaud, 1977; Renaud and Padjen, 1978; Renaud *et al.*, 1979; Wilber *et al.*, 1976), (5) its rapid degradation by brain peptidases (reviewed in Marks, 1977, 1978;

Table 5.17 Central actions of thyroliberin (adapted from Guillemin, 1978b).

Increases spontaneous motor activity
    Alters sleep patterns
    Produces anorexia
    Inhibits conditioned avoidance behavior
    Causes head to tail rotation

Opposes actions of barbiturates on sleeping time, hypothermia, and lethality
    Opposes actions of ethanol, chloral hydrate, chlorpromazine, and diazepam on
        sleeping time and hypothermia
    Enhances convulsion time and lethality of strychnine
    Increases motor activity in morphine-treated animals

Potentiates DOPA-pargyline effects

Ameliorates human behavioral disorders?

Causes central inhibition of morphine-mediated secretion of GH and PRL

Alters brain cell membrane electrical activity

Increases norepinephrine turnover
    Releases norepinephrine and dopamine from synaptosomal preparations
    Enhances disappearance of norepinephrine from nerve terminals

Potentiates excitatory actions of acetylcholine on cerebral cortical neurons

Winokur and Utiger, 1979), and (6) its binding to apparent receptor sites in brain, discussed in the next section.

5.6.2 Binding studies

The identification of high-affinity ^{3}H-TRH binding sites in the central nervous system as apparent receptors for TRH (Burt, 1978b, 1979; Burt and Snyder, 1975; Burt and Taylor, 1980) has depended in large part on comparison with pituitary receptors. Thus the identification of pituitary receptors will be considered initially.

High-affinity ^{3}H-TRH binding sites in various pituitary preparations have been identified as receptors for TRH largely on the basis of the excellent match between the relative potencies of TRH analogs in stimulating secretion of thyrotropin or prolactin and in inhibiting binding (Grant *et al.*, 1973a; Hinkle *et al.*, 1974; Vale *et al.*, 1973), although the specificity with respect to other hormones (Grant *et al.*, 1972; Labrie *et al.*, 1972), control cell strains (Hinkle and Tashjian, 1973), subcellular distribution (Poirier *et al.*, 1972) and other factors (discussed in Tixier-Vidal *et al.*, 1975) also contributed. Dissociation constants (K_Ds) for ^{3}H-TRH binding to pituitary membrane preparations at $0°C$ reported in these studies have ranged from 20 to 40 nM, exceeding the concentration of TRH required to stimulate thyrotropin or prolactin secretion half maximally at $37°C$ by 10- to 20-fold ('spare' receptors). For binding to intact GH$_3$ cells at $37°C$, half maximal binding occurs at 11 nM ^{3}H-TRH compared to half maximal stimulation of prolactin secretion at 2 nM TRH (Hinkle and Tashjian, 1973), i.e. the discrepancy is reduced but still present. The pharmacological properties of TRH receptors on prolactin-producing cells seem to be very similar or identical to those on thyrotropin-producing cells (Hinkle *et al.*, 1974). All authors agree that the initial binding step is largely reversible, although reported half-times of dissociation at $0°C$ have ranged from 1 to 3 min (Grant *et al.*, 1972) to 2 to 3 h (Hinkle and Tashjian, 1973).

The initial study of apparent brain receptors for TRH (Burt and Snyder, 1975), the first binding study for any neuropeptide in brain, started with a survey of rat tissues, looking for saturable binding of ^{3}H-TRH compared to a 1 mM TRH blank. Only 3 of 16 tissues examined showed appreciable binding: liver, which was higher than pituitary, pituitary, and whole brain, the lowest. Further examination showed that all of the binding to liver and most of the binding to brain was of relatively low affinity, about 5 μM, and thus presumably did not represent receptors. The low-affinity binding in brain was distinguishable from that in liver in its kinetic and other properties, however. A rather minor proportion of binding in brain, about 30 per cent of saturable binding and 15 per cent of total binding in rat cerebral cortex (Fig. 5.5), appeared to resemble pituitary binding in its

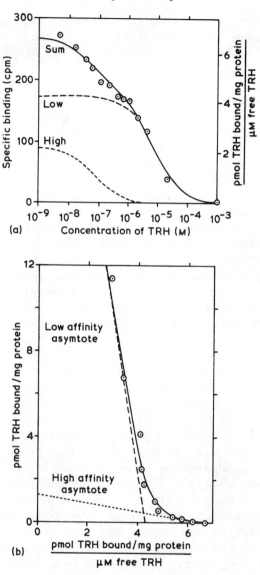

Fig. 5.5 Competition curve for binding of ^{3}H-TRH to membranes of rat cerebral cortex (a), and Scatchard plot of the results (b). The asymptotes of the Scatchard plot were used to derive the K_D and B_{max} for the low- and high-affinity sites as described in Burt and Snyder (1975). These values were used to express the original competition curve as the sum of curves representing the contribution of each type of site to the total binding. The blank in this experiment was 170 cpm. (Redrawn from Burt and Snyder, 1975.)

affinity, with apparent K_Ds of about 30 to 50 nM in various regions except cerebellum, where no high-affinity binding was detected. The cerebellum is also among the regions lowest in concentration of TRH-like immunore-activity (Jackson and Reichlin, 1974; Oliver *et al.*, 1974; Winokur and Utiger, 1974), although a proportion of cells do respond to iontophoretically applied TRH (Renaud and Martin, 1975).

Pharmacological studies showed a preference of the high-affinity binding only for [3-Me-His²]TRH over TRH. This analog also has about 8 to 10 times higher potency than TRH in the pituitary (Vale *et al.*, 1971). Later experiments have shown it to be about 10-fold more potent than TRH in inducing shaking movements by injection into the periaqueductal-fourth ventricular spaces of barbiturate-anesthetized rats (Wei *et al.*, 1976) and in depolarizing motoneurons in isolated frog spinal cord (Nicoll, 1977). Thus behavioral and electrophysiological measurements appeared to confirm the binding measurements in the pituitary-like preference of central TRH receptors for [3-Me-His²]TRH.

Unfortunately, further pharmacological and kinetic properties of the high-affinity ³H-TRH binding sites in rat brain were mostly obscured by the high blanks and the large excess of saturable but lower affinity sites, which themselves exhibited a considerable degree of pharmacological specificity (not unlike the pituitary). These technical difficulties discouraged further experimentation for several years.

The availability of ³H-TRH of higher specific activity in 1977–1978 encouraged another attempt to study central TRH receptors. The relative selectivity of [3-Me-His²]TRH for the high-affinity binding sites, observed in the initial study, meant that use of this analog in blank tubes (1 μM concentration) instead of TRH itself allowed selective observation of high-affinity sites as 'specific' binding. Low-affinity but saturable ³H-TRH binding was incorporated into the blanks along with non-saturable binding to filter and tissue, counting background, etc. Saturation and kinetic experiments thus could look exclusively at high-affinity binding, although competition experiments were still ambiguous, i.e. potentially seeing competition for both classes of binding sites.

Under these circumstances, and using membrane resuspensions at high concentrations (40 mg original wet weight/ml), rat forebrain yielded as much as 40 per cent specific binding, and rat spinal cord as much as 30 per cent (Burt, unpublished results). Spinal cord, not previously examined, had the advantage of relatively less saturable, low-affinity binding in the blanks. Table 5.18 shows a comparison of partial pharmacological properties of ³H-TRH binding in rat spinal cord and forebrain with those of binding in calf pituitary and published data in cell lines derived from rats. Both regions resembled each other and the pituitary, but the concentrations of high-affinity binding sites were very low, less than 1 pmol/g wet weight of

Table 5.18 IC_{50}s (nM) in competing for [^{3}H]TRH binding (Burt, unpublished results).

Analog	Pituitary cell lines (published)	Calf pituitary	Rat forebrain	Rat spinal cord
[3-Me-His^2]TRH (A-42872)	3* 4.7†	3.0 ± 0.3(5)	4.6 ± 1.0(3)	4.4 ± 0.5(3)
TRH (A-38579)	20* 25†	29 ± 5(7)	16 ± 4(3)	10 ± 2(3)
O=C < Thr-His-Pro-NH$_2$ (A-42347)	120†	240 ± 60(3)	130 ± 40(4)	100 ± 24(3)
O=C < Ser-His-Pro-NH$_2$ (A-42007)	200†	125 ± 25(2)	120 ± 30(3)	120 ± 35(3)
pGlu-His-Pro-NHET (A-42895)	600* 500†	870 ± 220(3)	210 ± 80(4)	500 ± 200(2)
10 other analogs	—	not tested	>10 000 on both regions	

* Grant *et al.* (1973a).
† Hinkle *et al.* (1974).
Data are means ± SEM for the indicated number of experiments.
All analogs were generously supplied by Dr A. M. Thomas of Abbott Laboratories.

tissue in both cases. This made studies of less potent analogs and kinetics of association and dissociation very difficult.

A phylogenetic survey, looking for better binding in lower vertebrates, detected little or no high-affinity ^{3}H-TRH binding to chicken brain, frog brain, or frog skin. All three tissues did have appreciable low-affinity binding ($K_D > 1$ μM).

The final and successful approach was to use a large mammalian brain, calf, sheep, or pig, from which relatively discrete smaller regions could be chosen and still have enough tissue to work with. A survey of a variety of brain regions in calf and sheep reported to have immunofluorescence for TRH in rat (Hökfelt *et al.*, 1975) yielded the best binding in the nucleus accumbens-septal area (Burt, 1978b; Burt and Taylor, 1980), with the specific binding about half of total binding. The nucleus accumbens is the area Hökfelt *et al.* (1975) reported to have the most dense TRH-like immunofluorescence outside the hypothalamus in rat. Kalivas and Horita (1979) recently reported the septum to be the area most sensitive to local application of TRH in antagonizing barbiturate narcosis. Both regions were routinely combined in order to get more tissue even though the nucleus accumbens appeared to have somewhat greater binding. Sheep brain was

Table 5.19 Comparison of parameters for ^{3}H-TRH binding to sheep anterior pituitary (PIT), nucleus accumbens-septal area (NA) and retina (RET) (data from Burt, 1979 and Burt and Taylor, 1980).

	PIT	NA	RET
$k_{-1}(\text{min}^{-1})$	$0.070 \pm 0.015(6)$	$0.074 \pm 0.004(2)$	$0.073 \pm 0.003(3)$
$k_1(\text{M}^{-1}\,\text{min}^{-1})$	$1.7 \pm 0.5(3)$ $\times 10^6$	$3.4 \pm 1.4(3)$ $\times 10^6$	$1.1 \pm 0.1(3)$ $\times 10^6$
$k_D = k_{-1}/k_1$ (nM)	41	22	66
K_D equilib (nM)	$43 \pm 9(6)$	$36 \pm 9(4)$	$35 \pm 8(5)$
B_{max}(pmol/g tiss.)	$20 \pm 4(6)$	$6 \pm 2(4)$	$5 \pm 1(5)$

chosen for further study because sheep pituitary gave better binding than calf or pig pituitary and had been used in the previous study (Burt and Snyder, 1975). Sheep retina was also tested because of the report by Schaeffer *et al.* (1977) that rat retina contains immunoreactive TRH whose levels increase after several hours of light. Sheep retinal ^{3}H-TRH binding was as good as that in the nucleus accumbens-septal area. Both regions were studied in detail and compared with sheep pituitary (Burt, 1978b, 1979; Burt and Taylor, 1980). A few experiments with rat retina also detected high-affinity ^{3}H-TRH binding, with an IC_{50} for TRH of about 18 nM and for [3-Me-His^2]TRH of about 5 nM (Burt, unpublished results).

   The kinetic and equilibrium properties of ^{3}H-TRH binding to sheep anterior pituitary, nucleus accumbens-septal area, and retina are compared in Table 5.19. It is evident on this basis that both central nervous system (CNS) regions are closely similar to each other and to the pituitary. A much more sensitive test of the similarity of the three tissues is comparison of their pharmacologies for competition by TRH analogs. Several analogs started competing for low-affinity binding sites in the CNS regions before the high-affinity sites. This was shown by their competition at concentrations slightly greater than their IC_{50}s being additive to the blanks, i.e. when the analog was added in combination with 1 μM [3-Me-His^2]TRH, binding was reduced below that observed with 1 μM [3-Me-His^2]TRH alone. Such analogs, for which unambiguous high-affinity IC_{50}s could not be obtained in the CNS regions, were excluded from the pharmacological comparisons illustrated in Figs. 5.6 and 5.7. The remaining 15 analogs, ranging over six orders of magnitude in potency, showed excellent agreement between their potencies in competing for CNS and pituitary binding sites. Even though the CNS data were relatively noisy because of high blanks, many possible systematic errors were prevented by running the comparisons in parallel with the same analog solutions, usually on the same day.

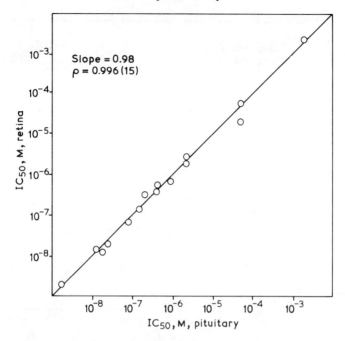

Fig. 5.6 Pharmacological comparison of high-affinity ^{3}H-TRH binding in sheep retina with that in sheep anterior pituitary. Mean IC$_{50}$s of 15 analogs are plotted against each other on a log–log scale. (Drawn from data tabulated in Burt, 1979.)

The binding data suggest that CNS TRH receptors are virtually identical to pituitary receptors in their pharmacology and in several other properties. Certain discrepancies have arisen between CNS and pituitary potencies of TRH analogs (Bissette *et al.*, 1978b; Breese *et al.*, 1975; Collu and Taché, 1979; Prange *et al.*, 1975; Veber *et al.*, 1977; and others), with many analogs appearing to show greater relative potencies in the CNS than their pituitary potencies would predict. When analogs are administered peripherally, greater lipophilicity and consequent greater ability to penetrate the blood–brain barrier could explain some enhanced effects in brain relative to pituitary. For central administration, increased resistance to brain peptidases could provide a similar explanation. It is not yet clear, however, that such factors can explain all apparent discrepancies, and it is possible that some central effects of TRH and its analogs, particularly at high doses, are mediated through less specific and perhaps lower affinity receptors which are distinct from the pituitary-like, high-affinity receptors.

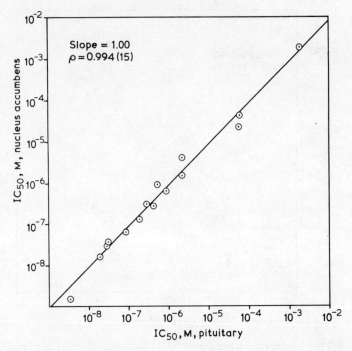

Fig. 5.7 Pharmacological comparison of high-affinity ^{3}H-TRH binding in sheep nucleus accumbens-septal area with that in sheep anterior pituitary. (Drawn from data tabulated in Burt and Taylor, 1980.)

5.6.3 Future directions

The apparent close similarity, and possible identity, of CNS receptor binding sites for TRH to pituitary receptors invites further exploration. Many advances that have been made in the regulation (Hinkle and Tashjian, 1975), solubilization (Hinkle and Lewis, 1978), visualization (Halpern and Hinkle, 1979), and mechanism of action (Labrie *et al.*, 1979) of pituitary TRH receptors may be applicable to brain receptors. The finding that TRH induces calcium-dependent action potentials in pituitary cells (Dufy *et al.*, 1979; Kidokoro, 1975; Taraskevich and Douglas, 1977) is especially interesting in trying to make analogies with possible mechanisms in nerve cells.

Binding studies of TRH receptors in brain will be greatly simplified by use of tritiated [3-Me-His^2]TRH as a higher affinity and more specific radioactive ligand (Taylor and Burt, 1980), but this is not yet generally available. Other technical advances in membrane purification or preparation, solubilization of receptors, or assay conditions also could lower blanks and simplify the assay.

Further exploration of the factors leading to dissociated CNS and pituitary potencies of certain TRH analogs will ultimately be necessary to determine whether the pituitary-like ^{3}H-TRH binding sites in brain are the receptors for all of TRH's central effects. Unfortunately, neither crude homogenates nor purified peptidase preparations (Dixon *et al.*, 1979; Hersh and McKelvy, 1979; Matsui *et al.*, 1979) may fully reflect the gauntlet run by released TRH or injected TRH or analogs on the way to its (their) receptor(s) in the intact brain. Thus full explanation of discrepancies may be difficult or impossible. The situation would be even more complicated if some of the central activities of TRH were due to a metabolite (Prasad *et al.*, 1977) rather than the intact tripeptide.

By studying the pharmacological interactions of TRH with other drugs and neurotransmitters, much evidence has been obtained that may bear on identifying neuronal systems which possess TRH receptors. Thus various central effects of TRH have been found to be blocked by atropine, naloxone, morphine, GABA agonists, etc. (see previously cited reviews). Other evidence has come from electrophysiological studies (e.g. Yarbrough, 1976) and studies of effects on neurotransmitter turnover or release (Malthe-Sørenssen *et al.*, 1978, reviewed in Horst *et al.*, 1979; Rastogi, 1979). It is likely that study of changes in receptor binding in response to lesions or disease or use of possible histochemical techniques for visualizing receptors, arising out of binding studies, also will have much to contribute to this area.

5.7 SOMATOSTATIN

5.7.1 Background

Somatostatin (SS, somatotropin release-inhibiting factor, H-Ala-Gly-Cys-Lys-Asn-Phe-Phe-Trp-Lys-Thr-Phe-Thr-Ser-Cys-OH) is a cyclic tetradecapeptide isolated from sheep hypothalami on the basis of its ability to inhibit the release of growth hormone by the anterior pituitary (Brazeau *et al.*, 1973). SS was soon found to inhibit the release of a variety of other hormones and other substances in the periphery (reviewed in Efendić *et al.*, 1978; Guillemin and Gerich 1976; Luft *et al.*, 1978; Vale *et al.*, 1977), including thyrotropin, glucagon, insulin, gastrin, gastric acid, secretin, VIP, renin, motilitin, cholecystokinin, pepsin, parathyroid hormone and calcitonin. SS-like immunoreactivity has been found to be correspondingly widely distributed in endocrine cells (A_1 or D cells) of the pancreas, gastrointestinal mucosa and thyroid and nerve cells and fibers of the autonomic nervous system, dorsal root (sensory) ganglia and central nervous system (reviewed in Elde *et al.*, 1978).

Three aspects of SS's distribution are particularly worthy of note. Its presence in small-diameter neurons of dorsal root ganglia and terminals in substantia gelatinosa of the dorsal horn of the spinal cord (Hökfelt *et al.*, 1976) makes it, along with substance P and possible angiotensin, a primary afferent transmitter candidate. Secondly, its presence in certain sympathetic neuronal cell bodies that are also capable of synthesizing catecholamines (Hökfelt *et al.*, 1977a) constitutes one of the earlier demonstrated possible contractions of Dale's principle. Finally, as in the case of TRH, most brain SS is extrahypothalamic (Brownstein *et al.*, 1975a; Kobayashi *et al.*, 1977), and lesion experiments suggest that most hypothalamic SS originates outside the hypothalamus (Brownstein *et al.*, 1977; Epelbaum *et al.*, 1977b). Table 5.20 gives the regional distribution of SS-like immunoreactivity in rat brain (Brownstein *et al.*, 1975a).

As might be expected from its wide distribution in the brain, SS has been reported to have a variety of behavioral and other central effects (reviewed in Kastin *et al.*, 1978). These include (Table 5.21) enhancement of the motor effects of L-dopa plus pargyline (Plotnikoff *et al.*, 1974), an effect produced more potently by TRH; enhancement of the sedative and hypothermic effects of barbiturates (Brown and Vale. 1975; Prange *et al.*, 1975), an effect opposite that of TRH; antagonism of the lethal effects of strychnine (Brown and Vale, 1975), an effect again opposite that of TRH; 'barrel' rotation (Cohn and Cohn, 1975); blockade of bombesin-induced hyperglycemia (Brown *et al.*, 1978c); analgesic effects, disturbances of sleep, generation of epileptic seizures, motor inco-ordination, akinesia and naloxone-insensitive, opiate-withdrawal-like symptoms (all reviewed in Havlicek and Friesen, 1979).

Table 5.20 Regional distribution of somatostatin in rat brain (Brownstein *et al.*, 1975a).

Region	ng/mg wet weight	ng/region
Olfactory bulb	0.02	1.0
Septum and preoptic area	0.64	24.7
Hypothalamus	2.12	39.3
Thalamus	0.15	17.5
Midbrain	0.06	9.5
Brain stem	0.05	9.8
Cerebellum	0.02	4.5
Striatum	0.05	3.2
Cortex	0.03	30.0

Table 5.21 Central actions of somatostatin.

Increased motor activity in dopa potentiation test.

Enhancement of pentobarbital sedation and hypothermia.

Antagonism of strychnine lethality.

'Barrel' rotation.

Blockade of bombesin-induced hyperglycemia.

Analgesic effects.

Disturbances of sleep.

Seizure activity.

Motor inco-ordination and akinesia.

'Wet dog shakes' and other opiate-withdrawal-like symptoms.

Reported *in vitro* actions of SS in brain include inhibition of release of TRH from organ-cultured hypothalamus (Hirooka *et al.*, 1978), enhancement of glutamate-induced uptake of and transient decrease in release of $^{45}C^{2+}$ in synaptosomes (Tan *et al.*, 1977), and enhancement of release of acetylcholine from hippocampal synaptosomes (Nemeth and Cooper, 1979). The effect on TRH, found in the 10^{-8} to 10^{-6} M range, resembles SS's effects on hormone secretion in the periphery, but the effect on acetylcholine is opposite to its reported effects in peripheral nerve (Guillemin, 1976). The effects on calcium and acetylcholine in synaptosomes should be interpreted with caution since both required SS concentrations in the micromolar range, whereas most peptide receptors have affinities in the low nanomolar range or lower.

Additional items of evidence suggest a possible neurotransmitter role of SS, or otherwise support the existence of SS receptors in brain. SS has a predominant synaptosomal localization in subcellular fractions of brain (Epelbaum *et al.*, 1977a). In response to depolarizing stimuli, it is released in a calcium-dependent manner from cell cultures of primary sensory neurons (Mudge *et al.*, 1977), from fragments of stalk median eminence or posterior pituitary (Patel *et al.*, 1978) and from slices of cerebral cortex (Havlicek and Friesen, 1979) and hypothalamus (Iversen *et al.*, 1978). There is preliminary evidence that it is synthesized in brain from larger precursors (Ensinck *et al.*, 1978; Spiess and Vale, 1978) and that it is rapidly inactivated by brain peptidases acting at several sites (Marks and Stern, 1975). Finally, iontophoretically applied SS inhibits firing of many neurons in various brain regions (Renaud *et al.*, 1975, 1976; Renaud and Padjen, 1978). In some cases SS may be excitatory (Dodd and Kelly, 1978).

5.7.2 Binding studies

This section will be necessarily brief since no full studies of possible SS receptors in brain have yet appeared. Preliminary demonstration of a degree of saturable binding of $[^{125}I\text{-}Tyr^1]SS$ or $[^{125}I\text{-}Tyr^1,D\text{-}Trp^3]SS$ to brain membranes (Lazarus, Perrin and Vale, unpublished) has been cited several times (Lazarus *et al.*, 1977a; Rivier *et al.*, 1976; Vale *et al.*, 1977), but the initial results were not promising enough to be worth following up (Vale, personal communication). The similarity of pituitary and brain receptor binding sites for TRH, already discussed, suggests that a brief review of the properties of pituitary receptors for SS may offer some guide to the properties to be expected of brain receptors.

The initial report (Schonbrunn and Tashjian, 1978) described binding of $[^{125}I\text{-}Tyr^1]SS$ to intact rat pituitary tumor cells (GH_4C_1 clonal strain) at 37° C under physiological conditions, so that the inhibition of growth hormone and prolactin secretion could be directly compared to binding. The K_D of the binding was 0.6 nM, k_1 was 8×10^7 M^{-1} min^{-1}, and k_{-1} was 0.02 to 0.04 min^{-1}. There was no comparative pharmacology of different SS analogs, but the authors were able to make an excellent case for identifying their binding with SS receptors both by the good agreement between the concentration dependence of inhibition of binding with that of inhibition of secretion for SS itself and by the correlation between presence of binding in 3 of 5 pituitary cell strains and presence of response to SS in the same 3 of 5 strains.

A second paper (Leitner *et al.*, 1979) described binding of $[^{125}I\text{-}Tyr^1]SS$ to a plasma membrane fraction from bovine anterior pituitaries. Samples were incubated for 18 h at 4° C and bound radioactivity was separated by alcohol precipitation and centrifugation. Binding was resolved into two components of apparent K_Ds of 30 nM and 8 μM. $[D\text{-}Trp^8]SS$ was observed to be about equal in potency to SS as an inhibitor of binding, while $[Ala^8]SS$ was considerably less potent. The former analog has enhanced activity compared to SS in many systems, while the latter is essentially inactive. Although results with these two analogs thus agree fairly well with expectations, disturbing factors are the high blanks and the relatively low affinity of the binding compared to results in pituitary tumor cells and compared to receptor binding of most other peptides of comparable size. The initial report is thus probably a better guide to expected properties of possible brain receptors for SS.

With the exception of an earlier report of relatively low-affinity binding of $[^{125}I\text{-}Tyr^1]SS$ by a widely distributed soluble protein (Ogawa *et al.*, 1977), the above two papers on pituitary are the only descriptions of possible SS receptor binding in any tissue. In addition, this author (Burt, unpublished results) has observed a low and variable degree of saturable binding of $[^{125}I\text{-}Tyr^1]SS$ to membranes of rat pancreas. Technical problems with high blanks have hindered progress in this area, but it is hoped they will eventually be overcome.

5.7.3 Future directions

Much effort has been devoted to developing SS analogs with selective effects on glucagon secretion for possible use in diabetes. Much progress has been made using *in vitro* and *in vivo* bioassays (Brown *et al.*, 1977c; Vale *et al.*, 1978), but understanding of the extent to which possible receptor differences, as opposed to access differences and other factors, contribute to differences in response to various analogs would be greatly advanced by the introduction of receptor binding assays in the responding tissues, including brain. Binding assays for SS receptors in brain thus could help prevent SS's central effects appearing as undesirable side effects of clinical use of SS analogs that happen to penetrate the blood–brain barrier.

On a more basic level, the availability of SS receptor binding assays in brain could materially advance knowledge of the mechanisms of SS's actions in the CNS, helping answer such questions as whether SS's inhibition of hormone secretion is related in mechanism to SS's inhibition of neuronal firing and whether SS receptors are presynaptic or postsynaptic or both. It would also help determine whether recently developed brain-selective SS analogs (Brown *et al.*, 1979) have higher affinity for brain receptors than others or whether their marked hydrophobicity can account in full for this effect.

5.8 CONCLUDING REMARKS

The choice of which six 'other peptides' to cover in this chapter has been rather arbitrary. Additional peptides with claims as possible neurotransmitters, neuromodulators or neurohormones, and for which receptors have been partially characterized in some tissue, include carnosine (Hirsch *et al.*, 1978), luliberin (Dyer and Dyball, 1974; Grant *et al.*, 1973b; Jan *et al.*, 1979; Moss *et al.*, 1979), vasopressin (Bockaert *et al.*, 1973; DeWied *et al.*, 1975a), oxytocin (Nilaver *et al.*, 1978; Soloff *et al.*, 1973; Swanson, 1978), bradykinin (Corrêa and Graeff, 1975; Corrêa *et al.*, 1978), cholecystokinin octapeptide (Dockray, 1976; Gardner, 1979), corticotropin (DeWied *et al.*, 1975b, Krieger *et al.*, 1977; Lefkowitz *et al.*, 1970) and prolactin (Clemens *et al.*, 1971, Fuxe *et al.*, 1977a; Shiu and Friesen, 1974). No doubt many additional candidates wait to be found.

REFERENCES

Almquist, S. (1972), *Front. Horm. Res.*, **1**, 38–47.
Anastasi, A., Erspamer, V. and Bucci, M. (1971), *Experientia*, **27**, 166–167.
Andersson, B. (1978), *Physiol. Rev.*, **58**, 582–603.
Andersson, S., Chang, D., Folkers, K. and Rosell, S. (1976), *Life Sci.*, **19**, 367–370.
Arregui, A., Bennett, J.P. Jr, Bird, E.D., Yamamura, H.I., Iversen, L.L. and Snyder, S.H. (1977), *Ann. Neurol.*, **2**, 294–298.
Barnea, A., Oliver, C. and Porter, J.C. (1977), in: *Hypothalamic Hormones and Pituitary Regulation*. (Porter, J.C., ed), Plenum Press, New York, pp. 49–75.
Bennett, J.P. Jr and Snyder, S.H. (1976), *J. biol. Chem.*, **251**, 7423–7430.
Bennett, J.P. Jr and Snyder, S.H. (1980), *Eur. J. Pharmacol.*, in press.
Bertaccini, G. (1976), *Pharmacol. Rev.*, **28**, 127–177.
Besson, J., Rotsztehn, W., Laburthe, M., Epelbaum, J., Beaudet, A., Kordon, K. and Rosselin, G. (1979), *Brain Res.*, **165**, 79–85.
Bissette, G., Manberg, P., Nemeroff, C.B. and Prange, A.J. Jr (1978a), *Life Sci.*, **23**, 2173–2182.
Bissette, G., Nemeroff, C.B., Loosen, P.T., Breese, G.R., Burnett, G.B., Lipton, M.A. and Prange, A.J. Jr (1978b), *Neuropharmacology*, **17**, 229–237.
Bissette, G., Nemeroff, C.B., Loosen, P.T., Prange, A.J. Jr and Lipton, M.A. (1976), *Nature*, **262**, 607–609.
Bockaert, J., Roy, C., Rajerison, R. and Jard, S. (1973), *J. biol. Chem.*, **248**, 5922–5931.
Borghi, C., Nicosia, S., Giachetti, A. and Said, S.I. (1979), *Life Sci.*, **24**, 65–70.
Brazeau, P., Vale, W., Burgus, R., Ling, N., Butcher, M., Rivier, J. and Guillemin, R. (1973), *Science*, **179**, 77–79.
Breese, G.R., Cott, J.M., Cooper, B.R., Prange, A.J. Jr, Lipton, M.A. and Plotnikoff, N.P. (1975), *J. Pharmacol. exp. Ther.*, **193**, 11–22.
Brown, M., Allen, R., Villarreal, J., Rivier, J. and Vale, W. (1978a), *Life Sci.*, **23**, 2721–2728.
Brown, M., Rivier, J., Kobayashi, R. and Vale, W. (1978b), in: *Gut Hormones*. (Bloom, S.R., ed), Churchill Livingstone, Edinburgh, pp. 550–558.
Brown, M., Rivier, J. and Vale, W. (1977a), *Science*, **196**, 998–1000.
Brown, M.R., Rivier, J. and Vale, W.W. (1977b), *Life Sci.*, **21**, 1729–1734.
Brown, M., Rivier, J. and Vale, W. (1977c), *Science*, **196**, 1467–1469.
Brown, M., Rivier, J. and Vale, W. (1977d), *Life Sci.*, **20**, 1681–1688.
Brown, M., Rivier, J. and Vale, W. (1978c), *Metabolism*, **27**, (Suppl. 1), 1253–1256.
Brown, M., Rivier, J. and Vale, W. (1979), *Endocrinology*, **104**, 1709–1715.
Brown, M. and Vale, W. (1975), *Endocrinology*, **96**, 1333–1336.
Brown, M.R. and Vale, W. (1976), *Endocrinology*, **98**, 819–822.
Brown, M. and Vale, W. (1979), *Trends in Neurosciences*, **2**, 95–97.
Brownstein, M.J., Arimura, A., Fernandez-Durango, R., Schally, A.V. and Kizer, J.S. (1977), *Endocrinology*, **100**, 246–249.
Brownstein, M., Arimura, A., Sato, M., Schally, A.V. and Kizer, J.S. (1975a), *Endocrinology*, **96**, 1456–1461.

Brownstein, M.J., Utiger, R.D., Palkovits, M. and Kizer, J.S. (1975b), *Proc. natn. Acad. Sci. USA,* **72**, 4177–4179.

Bryant, M.G., Bloom, S.R., Polak, J.M., Albuquerque, R.H., Modlin, I. and Pearse, A.G.E. (1976), *Lancet,* **i**, 991–993.

Buckley, J.P. (1977), *Biochem. Pharmacol.,* **26**, 1–3.

Buffa, R, Capella, C., Solcia, E., Feigerio, B. and Said, S.I. (1977), *Histochemistry,* **50**, 217–227.

Burgus, R., Dunn, T.F., Desiderio, D., Ward, D.N., Vale, W. and Guillemin, R. (1970), *Nature,* **226**, 321–325.

Burt, D.R. (1978a), in: *Neurotransmitter Receptor Binding.* (Yamamura, H.I., Enna, S.J. and Kuhar, M.J., eds), Raven Press, New York, pp. 41–55.

Burt, D.R. (1978b), *Neuroscience Abs.,* **4**, 406 (Abs. No. 1277).

Burt, D.R. (1979), *Exp. Eye Res.,* **29**, 353–365.

Burt, D.R. and Snyder, S.H. (1975), *Brain Res.,* **93**, 309–328.

Burt, D.R. and Taylor, R.L. (1980), *Endocrinology,* **106**, 1416–1423.

Carraway, R. and Leeman, S.E. (1973), *J. biol. Chem.,* **248**, 6854–6861.

Carraway, R. and Leeman, S.E. (1975a), *J. biol. Chem.,* **250**, 1907–1911.

Carraway, R. and Leeman, S.E. (1975b), in: *Peptides: Chemistry, Structure and Biology.* (Walter, R. and Meinhofer, J., eds), Ann Arbor Science Publishers, Ann Arbor, Michigan, pp. 679–685.

Carraway, R. and Leeman, S.E. (1976a), *J. biol. Chem.,* **251**, 7035–7044.

Carraway, R. and Leeman, S.E. (1976b), *J. biol. Chem.,* **251**, 7045–7052.

Changaris, P.G., Keil, L.C. and Severs, W.B. (1978), *Neuroendocrinology,* **25**, 257–274.

Clark, W.G., Lipton, J.M. and Said, S.I. (1978), *Neuropharmacol.,* **17**, 883–885.

Clemens, J.A., Gallo, R.V., Whitmoyer, D.I. and Sawyer, C.H. (1971), *Brain Res.,* **25**, 371–379.

Clineschmidt, B.V. and McGuffin, J.C. (1977), *Eur. J. Pharmacol.,* **46**, 395–396.

Clineschmidt, B.V., McGuffin, J.C. and Bunting, P.B. (1979), *Eur. J. Pharmacol.,* **54**, 129–139.

Cohn, M.L. and Cohn, M. (1975), *Brain Res.,* **96**, 138–141.

Cole, F.E., Frohlich, E.D. and Macphee, A.A. (1978), *Brain Res.,* **154**, 178–181.

Collu, R. and Taché, Y. (1979), in: *Central Nervous System Effects of Hypothalamic Hormones and Other Peptides.* (Collu, R., Barbeau, A., Ducharme, J.R. and Rochefort, J.G., eds), Raven Press, New York, pp. 97–121.

Corrêa, F.M.A. and Graeff, F.G. (1975), *J. Pharmacol. exp. Therm.,* **192**, 670–676.

Corrêa, F.M.A., Innis, R.B. and Snyder, S.H. (1978), *Neuroscience Abs.,* **4**, 406 (Abs. No. 1280).

Cuatrecasas, P. (1976), in: *Pre and Postsynaptic Receptors.* (Usdin, E. and Bunney, W.E., eds), Marcel Dekker, New York, pp. 245–264.

Deschodt-Lanckman, M., Robberecht, P. and Christophe, J. (1977), *FEBS Letters,* **83**, 76–80.

Devynck, M.A. and Meyer, P. (1978), *Biochem. Pharmacol.,* **27**, 1–5.

De Wied, D., Bohus, B. and van Wimersman Greidanus, T.B. (1975a), *Brain Res.,* **85**, 152–156.

De Wied, D., Witter, A. and Greven, H.M. (1975b), *Biochem. Pharm.,* **24**, 1463–1468.

Dixon, J.E., Rupnow, J.H., Taylor, W.L. and Andrews, P.C. (1979), *Fed. Proc.*, **38**, 350 (Abs. No. 639).

Dockray, G.J. (1976), *Nature*, **264**, 568–57C.

Dodd, J. and Kelly, J.S. (1978), *Nature*, **273**, 674–675.

Dufy, B., Vincent, J.-D., Fleury, H., DuPasquier, P., Gourdji, D. and Tixier-Vidal, A. (1979), *Science*, **204**, 509–511.

Dupont, A. and Mérand, Y. (1978), *Life Sci.*, **22**, 1623–1630.

Dyer, R.G. and Dyball, R.E.J. (1974), *Nature*, **252**, 486–488.

Efendić, S., Hökfelt, T. and Luft, R. (1978), *Adv. metab. Disord.*, **9**, 367–424.

Elde, R., Hökfelt, T., Johansson, O., Schultzberg, M., Efendić, S. and Luft, R. (1978), *Metabolism*, **27** (Suppl. 1), 1151–1159.

Emson, P.C., Fahrenkrug, J., Schaffalitzky de Muckadell, O.B., Jessel, T.M. and Iversen, L.L. (1978), *Brain Res.*, **143**, 174–178.

Ensinck, J.W., Laschansky, E.C., Kanter, R.A., Fujimoto, W. Y., Koerker, D.J. and Goodner, C.J. (1978), *Metabolism*, **27** (Suppl. 1), 1207–1210.

Epelbaum, J., Brazeau, P., Tsang, D., Brawer, D. and Martin, J.B. (1977a), *Brain Res.*, **126**, 309–323.

Epelbaum, J., Tapia-Arancibia, L., Rotsztejn, W., Besson, J. and Kordon, C. (1979), *Proc. endocrine Soc.*, 61st Meet., p. 145 (Abs. No. 289).

Epelbaum, J., Willoughby, J.O., Brazeau, P. and Martin, J.B. (1977b), *Endocrinology*, **101**, 1495–1502.

Epstein, A.N. (1978), in: *Frontiers in Neuroendocrinology*, Vol. 5. (Ganong, W.F. and Martini, L., eds), Raven Press, New York, pp. 101–134.

Erspamer, V. and Melchiorri, P. (1973), *Pure appl. Chem.*, **35**, 463–494.

Erspamer, V. and Melchiorri, P. (1975), in: *Gastrointestinal Hormones.* (Thompson, J.C., ed), University of Texas, Austin, pp. 575–589.

Escher, E.H., Nguyen, T.M., Robert, H., St. Pierre, S.A. and Rigoli, D.C. (1978), *J. med. Chem.*, **21**, 860–864.

Felix, D. and Schlegel, W. (1978), *Brain Res.*, **149**, 107–116.

Ferrario, C.M., Gildenberg, P.L. and McCubbin, J.W. (1972), *Circ. Res.*, **30**, 257–262.

Fitzsimons, J.T., Epstein, A.N. and Johnson, A.K. (1978), *Brain Res.*, **153**, 319–331.

Fuxe, K., Ganten, D., Hökfelt, T. and Bolme, P. (1976), *Neurosci. Lett.*, **2**, 229–234.

Fuxe, K., Hökfelt, T., Eneroth, P., Gustafsson, J.A. and Skett, P. (1977a), *Science*, **196**, 899–900.

Fuxe, K., Hökfelt, T., Said, S.I. and Mutt, V. (1977b), *Neurosci. Lett.*, **5**, 241–246.

Ganten, D., Fuxe, K., Phillips, M.I., Mann, J.F.E. and Ganten, U. (1978), in: *Frontiers in Neuroendocrinology*, Vol. 5. (Ganong, W.F. and Martini, L., eds), Raven Press, New York, pp. 61–99.

Ganten, D. and Speck, G. (1978), *Biochem. Pharmacol.*, **27**, 2379–2389.

Garcia-Sevilla, J.A., Magnusson, T., Carlsson, A., Leban, J. and Folkers, K. (1978), *Naunyn-Schmideberg's Arch. Pharmacol.*, **305**, 213–218.

Gardner, J.D. (1979), *Gastroenterology*, **76**, 202–214.

Giachetti, A., Said, S.I., Reynolds, R.C. and Koniges, F.C. (1977), *Proc. natn. Acad. Sci. USA*, **74**, 3424–3428.

Grant, G., Vale, W. and Guillemin, R. (1972), *Biochem. biophys. Res. Commun.*, **46**, 28–34.

Grant, G., Vale, W. and Guillemin, R. (1973a), *Endocrinology,* **92**, 1629–1633.
Grant, G., Vale, W. and Rivier, J. (1973b), *Biochem. biophys. Res. Commun.,* **50**, 771–778.
Grimm-Jørgensen, Y., McKelvy, J.F. and Jackson, I.M.D. (1975), *Nature,* **254**, 620.
Guillemin, R. (1976), *Endocrinology,* **99**, 1653–1654.
Guillemin, R. (1978a), *Science,* **202**, 390–402.
Guillemin, R. (1978b), in: *The Hypothalamus.* (Reichlin, S., Baldessarini, R.J. and Martin, J.B., eds), Raven Press, New York, pp. 155–194.
Guillemin, R. and Gerich, J.E. (1976), *Ann. Rev. Med.,* **27**, 379–388.
Halpern, J. and Hinkle, P.M. (1979), *Proc. endocrine Soc.,* 61st Meet., p. 178 (Abs. No. 421).
Havlicek, V. and Friesen, H. (1979), in: *Central Nervous System Effects of Hypothalamic Hormones and Other Peptides.* (Collu, R., Barbeau, A., Ducharme, J.D. and Rochefort, J.-G., eds), Raven Press, New York, pp. 381–402.
Hersh, L.B. and McKelvy, J.F. (1979), *Brain Res.,* **168**, 553–564.
Hinkle, P.M. and Lewis, D. (1978), *Biochem. biophys. Acta,* **541**, 347–359.
Hinkle, P.M. and Tashjian, A.H. Jr (1973), *J. biol. Chem.,* **248**, 6180–6186.
Hinkle, P.M. and Tashjian, A.H. Jr (1975), *Biochemistry,* **14**, 3845–3851.
Hinkle, P.M., Woroch, E.L. and Tashjian, A.H. Jr (1974), *J. biol. Chem.,* **249**, 3085–3090.
Hirooka, Y., Hollander, C.S., Suzuki, S., Ferdinand, P. and Juan, S.-I. (1978), *Proc. natn. Acad. Sci. USA,* **75**, 4509–4513.
Hirsch, J.D., Grille, M. and Margolis, F.L. (1978), *Brain Res.,* **158**, 407–422.
Hoffman, W.E., Phillips, M.I. and Schmid, P.G. (1977a), *Am. J. Physiol.,* **232**, H426–H433.
Hoffman, W.E., Phillips, M.I., Schmid, P.G., Falcon, J. and Weet, J.F. (1977b), *Neuropharmacol.,* **16**, 463–472.
Hökfelt, T., Elde, R., Johansson, O., Luft, R., Nilsson, G. and Arimura, A. (1976), *Neuroscience,* **1**, 131–136.
Hökfelt, T., Elfvin, L.G., Elde, R., Schultzberg, M., Goldstein, M. and Luft, R. (1977a), *Proc. natn. Acad. Sci. USA,* **74**, 3587–3591.
Hökfelt, T., Elfvin, L.G., Schultzberg, M., Fuxe, K., Said, S.I., Mutt, V. and Goldstein, M. (1977b), *Neuroscience,* **2**, 885–896.
Hökfelt, T., Fuxe, K., Johansson, O., Jeffcoate, S. and White, N. (1975), *Eur. J. Pharmacol.,* **34**, 389–392.
Horita, A., Carino, M.A., Lai, H. and La Hann, T.R. (1979), in: *Central Nervous System Effects of Hypothalamic Hormones and Other Peptides.* (Collu, R., Barbeau, A., Ducharme, J.R. and Rochefort, J.G., eds), Raven Press, New York, pp. 65–74.
Horst, W.D., Spirt, N. and Bautz, G. (1979), in: *Central Nervous System Effects of Hypothalamic Hormones and Other Peptides.* (Collu, R., Barbeau, A., Ducharme, J.R. and Rochefort, J.G., eds), Raven Press, New York, pp. 141–143.
Iversen, L.L., Iversen, S.D., Bloom, F., Douglas, C., Brown, M. and Vale, W. (1978), *Nature,* **273**, 161–163.
Jackson, I.M.D. (1978), *Am. Zool.,* **18**, 385–399.

Jackson, I.M.D. and Reichlin, S. (1974), *Endocrinology,* **95**, 854–862.

Jackson, I.M.D. and Reichlin, S. (1979), in: *Central Nervous System Effects of Hypothalamic Hormones and Other Peptides.* (Collu, R., Barbeau, A., Ducharme, J.R. and Rochefort, J.G., eds), Raven Press, New York, pp. 3–54.

Jan, Y.N., Jan, L.Y. and Kuffler, S.W. (1979), *Proc. natn. Acad. Sci. USA,* **76,** 1501–1505.

Jensen, R.I., Moody, T., Pert, C., Rivier, J.E. and Gardner, J.D. (1978), *Proc. natn. Acad. Sci. USA,* **75,** 6139–6143.

Kalivas, P.W. and Horita, A. (1979), *Nature,* **278,** 461–463.

Kastin, A.J., Coy, D.H., Jacquet, Y., Schally, A.V. and Plotnikoff, N.P. (1978), *Metabolism,* **27** (Suppl. 1), 1247–1252.

Kato, Y., Iwasaki, Y., Iwasaki, J., Abe, H., Yanaihara, N. and Imura, H. (1978), *Endocrinology,* **103,** 554–558.

Khosla, M.C., Smeby, R.R. and Bumpus, F.M. (1974), in: *Angiotensin, Handbook of Experimental Pharmacology,* Vol. 37. (Page, I.H. and Bumpus, F.M., eds), Springer-Verlag, New York, pp. 126–161.

Kidokoro, Y. (1975), *Nature,* **258,** 741–742.

Kitabgi, P., Carraway, R., Van Rietschoten, J., Granier, C., Morgat, J.L., Menez, A., Leeman, S. and Freychet, P. (1977), *Proc. natn. Acad. Sci. USA,* **74,** 1846–1850.

Kitabgi, P. and Freychet, P. (1979), *Eur. J. Pharmacol.,* **55,** 35–42.

Klotz, I.M and Hunston, D.L. (1971), *Biochemistry,* **10,** 3065–3069.

Kobayashi, R.M., Brown, M. and Vale, W. (1977), *Brain Res.,* **126,** 584–588.

Krieger, D.T., Liotta, A. and Brownstein, M.J. (1977), *Proc. natn. Acad. Sci. USA,* **74,** 648–652.

Labrie, F., Barden, N., Poirier, G. and De Lean, A. (1972), *Proc. natn. Acad. Sci. USA,* **69,** 283–387.

Labrie, F., Borgeat, P., Drouin, J., Beaulieu, M., Lagace, L., Ferland, L. and Raymond, V. (1979), *Ann. Rev. Physiol.,* **41,** 555–569.

Larsson, L.-I. (1977), *Histochemistry,* **54,** 173–176.

Larsson, L.I., Edvinsson, L., Fahrenkrug, J., Håkanson, R., Owman, C., Schaffalitzky de Muckadell, O. and Sundler, F. (1976a), *Brain Res.,* **13,** 400–404.

Larsson, L.I., Edvinsson, L., Fahrenkrug, J., Schaffalitzky de Muckadell, O.B., Sundler, F., Håkanson, R. and Rehfeld, J.F. (1976b), *Proc. natn. Acad. Sci. USA,* **73,** 3197–3200.

Larsson, L.I., Fahrenkrug, J. and Schaffalitzky de Muckadell, O.B. (1977), *Science,* **197,** 1374–1375.

Lazarus, L.H., Brown, M.R. and Perrin, M.H. (1977a), *Neuropharmacology,* **16,** 625–629.

Lazarus, L.H., Perrin, M.H. and Brown, M.R. (1977b), *J. biol. Chem.,* **252,** 7174–7179.

Lefkowitz, R.J., Roth, J., Pricer, W. and Pastan, F. (1970), *Proc. natn. Acad. Sci. USA,* **65,** 745–752.

Leitner, J.W., Rifkin, R.M., Maman, A. and Sussman, K.E. (1979), *Biochem. biophys. Res. Commun.,* **87,** 919–927.

Loosen, P.T., Nemeroff, C.B., Bissette, G., Burnett, G.B., Prange, A.J. Jr and
    Lipton, M.A. (1978), *Neuropharmacology*, **17**, 109–113.
Luft, R., Efendic, S. and Hökfelt, T. (1978), *Diabetologia*, **14**, 1–13.
Malthe-Sørenssen, D., Wood, P.L., Cheney, D.L. and Costa, E. (1978),
    J. Neurochem., **31**, 685–691.
Marks, N. (1977), in: *Peptides in Neurobiology*. (Gainer, H., ed), Plenum Press, New
    York, pp. 221–258.
Marks, N. (1978), in: *Frontiers in Neuroendocrinology*, Vol. 5, (Ganong, W.F. and
    Martini, L., eds), Raven Press, New York, pp. 329–377.
Marks, N. and Stern, F. (1975), *FEBS Letters*, **55**, 220–224.
Martino, E., Lernmark, A., Seo, H., Steiner, D.F. and Refetoff, S. (1978), *Proc.
    natn. Acad. Sci. USA*, **75**, 4265–4267.
Matsui, T., Prasad, C. and Peterkofsky, A. (1979), *J. biol. Chem.*, **254**,
    2439–2445.
McKelvy, J.F. and Epelbaum, J. (1978), in: *The Hypothalamus*. (Reichlin, S.,
    Baldessarini, R.J. and Martin, J.B., eds), Raven Press, New York,
    pp. 195–211.
Melchiorri, P. (1978), in: *Gut Hormones*. (Bloom, S.R., ed), Churchill Livingstone,
    Edinburgh, pp. 534–540.
Miletic, V. and Randic, M. (1978), *Neuroscience Abs.*, **4**, 411 (Abs. No. 1300).
Mogenson, G.J. and Kucharczyk, J. (1978), *Federation Proc.*, **37**, 2683–2688.
Moody, T.W., Pert, C.B., Rivier, J. and Brown, M.R. (1978), *Proc. natn. Acad. Sci.
    USA*, **75**, 5372–5376.
Morely, J.E., Garvin, T.J., Pekary, A.E. and Hershman, J.M. (1977), *Biochem.
    biophys. Res. Comm.*, **79**, 314–318.
Morley, J.E., Levin, S.R., Pehlevanian, M., Adachi, A., Pekary, E. and Hershman,
    J.M. (1979a), *Endocrinology*, **104**, 137–139.
Morely, J.E., Steinbach, J.H., Feldman, E.J. and Solomon, T.E. (1979b), *Life Sci.*,
    24, 1059–1066.
Moss, R.L., Riskind, P. and Dudley, C.A. (1979), in: *Central Nervous System Effects
    of Hypothalamic Hormones and Other Peptides*. (Collu, R., Barbeau, A.,
    Ducharme, J. and Rochefort, J.-G., eds), Raven Press, New York,
    pp. 345–366.
Mudge, A.W., Fishback, G.D. and Leeman, S.E. (1977), *Neurosci. Abs.*, **3**, 410
    (Abs. No. 1306).
Nahmod, V.E., Finkielman, S., de Gorodner, O.S. and Goldstein, D.J. (1977), in:
    Central Actions of Angiotensin and Related Hormones. (Buckley, J.P. and
    Ferrario, C., eds), Pergamon Press, New York, pp. 573–578.
Nair, R.M. G., Barrett, J.F., Bowers, C.Y. and Schally, A.V. (1970), *Biochemistry*, **9**,
    1103–1106.
Nemeroff, C.B., Bissette, G., Manberg, P.J., Osbahr, A.J. III, Breese, G.R., Loosen,
    P.T., Lipton, M.A. and Prange, A.J. Jr (1978), *Neuroscience Abs.*, **4**, 412
    (Abs. No. 1302).
Nemeroff, C.B., Bissette, G., Prange, A.J. Jr, Loosen, P.T., Barlow, T.S. and Lipton,
    M.A. (1977), *Brain Res.*, **128**, 485–496.
Nemeth, E.F. and Cooper, J.R. (1979), *Brain Res.*, **165**, 166–170.
Nicoll, R.A. (1977), *Nature*, **265**, 242–243.

Nilaver, G., Wilkins, J., Michaels, J., Hoffman, D.L., Silverman, A.J. and Zimmerman, E.A. (1978), *Neuroscience Abs.,* **4**, 351 (Abs. No. 1118).

Ogawa, N., Thompson, T., Friesen, H.G., Martin, J.B. and Brazeau, P. (1977), *Biochem. J.,* **165**, 269–277.

Oliver, C., Eskay, R.L., Ben-Jonathan, N. and Porter, J.C. (1974), *Endocrinology,* **95**, 540–546.

Osbahr, A.J. III, Nemeroff, C.B., Manberg, P.J. and Prange, A.J. Jr (1979), *Eur. J. Pharmacol.,* **54**, 299–302.

Patel, Y.C., Zingg, H.H. and Dreifuss, J.J. (1978), *Metabolism,* **27**, Suppl. 1, 1243–1245.

Peach, M.J. (1977), *Physiol. Rev.,* **57**, 313–370.

Peach, M.J. (1979), *Kidney Internat.,* **15**, S3–S6.

Pearse, A.G.E. (1976), *Nature,* **262**, 92–94.

Pearse, A.G.E. (1978), in: *Centrally Acting Peptides.* (Hughes, J., ed), University Park Press, Baltimore, pp. 49–57.

Phillips, M.I. (1978a), *Neuroendocrinology,* **25**, 354–377.

Phillips, I. (1978b), in: *Nervous System and Hypertension.* (Schmitt, H. and Meyer, P., eds), John Wiley and Son, New York, pp. 102–105.

Phillips, M. I. and Felix, D. (1976), *Brain Res.,* **109**, 531–540.

Phillips, M.I., Felix, D., Hoffman, W.E. and Ganten, D. (1977a), in: *Approaches to the Cell Biology of Neurons.* (Cowan, W.M. and Ferrendelli, J.A., eds), Society for Neuroscience, Bethesda, Maryland, pp. 308–339.

Phillips, M.I., Mann, J.F.E., Haebara, H., Hoffman, W.E., Dietz, R., Schelling, P. and Ganten, D. (1977b), *Nature,* **270**, 445–447.

Phillis, J.W., Kirkpatrick, J.R. and Said, S.I. (1978), *Can. J. Physiol. Pharmacol.,* **56**, 337–340.

Plotnikoff, N.P., Kastrin, A.J. and Schally, A.V. (1974), *Pharmacol. Biochem. Behav.,* **2**, 693–696.

Poirier, G., Labrie, F., Barden, N. and Lemaire, S. (1972), *FEBS Lett.,* **20**, 283–286.

Polak, J.M., Buchan, A.M.J., Czykowska, W., Solcia, E., Bloom, S.R. and Pearse, A.G.E. (1978), in: *Gut Hormones.* (Bloom, S.R., ed), Churchill Livingstone, Edinburgh, pp. 541–543.

Polak, J.M., Pearse, A.G.E., Garaud, J.C. and Bloom, S.R. (1974), *Gut,* **15**, 720–724.

Polak, J.M., Sullivan, S.N., Bloom, S.R., Buchan, A.M.J., Facer, P., Brown, M.R. and Pearse, A.G.E. (1977), *Nature,* **270**, 183–184.

Porter, J.C., Eskay, R.L., Oliver, C., Ben-Jonathan, N., Warberg, J., Parker, C.R. Jr. and Barnea, A. (1977), in: *Hypothalamic Hormones and Pituitary Regulation.* (Porter, J.C., ed), Plenum Press, New York, pp. 181–201.

Prange, A.J. Jr, Breese, G.R., Jahnke, G.D., Martin, B.R., Cooper, B.R., Cott, J.M., Wilson, I.C., Alltop, L.B., Lipton, M.A., Bissette, G., Nemeroff, C.F. and Loosen, P.T. (1975), *Life Sci.,* **16**, 1907–1914.

Prange, A.J. Jr, Nemeroff, C.B. and Lipton, M.A. (1978a), in: *Psychopharmacology: A Generation of Progress.* (Lipton, M.A., Di Mascio, A. and Killam, K.F., eds), Raven Press, New York, pp. 441–458.

Prange, A.J. Jr, Nemeroff, C.B., Lipton, M.A., Breese, G.R. and Wilson, I.C.

(1978b), in: *Handbook of Psychopharmacology,* Vol. 13. (Iversen, L.L., Iversen, S.D. and Snyder, S.H., eds), Plenum Press, New York, pp. 1–107.

Prange, A.J. Jr, Nemeroff, C.B. and Loosen, P.T. (1978c), in: *Centrally Acting Peptides.* (Hughes, J., ed), University Park Press, Baltimore, pp. 99–118.

Prange, A.J. Jr, Nemeroff, C.B., Loosen, P.T., Bissette, G., Osbahr, A. III, Wilson, I.C. and Lipton, M.S. (1979), in: *Central Nervous System Effects of Hypothalamic Hormones and Other Peptides.* (Collu, R., Barbeau, A., Ducharme, J.R. and Rochefort, J.-G., eds), Raven Press, New York, pp. 75–96.

Prasad, C., Matsui, T. and Peterkofsky, A. (1977), *Nature,* **268**, 142–144.

Rastogi, R.B. (1979), in: *Central Nervous System Effects of Hypothalamic Hormones and Other Peptides.* (Collu, R., Barbeau, A., Ducharme, J.R. and Rochefort, J.G., eds), Raven Press, New York, pp. 123–140.

Regoli, D., Park, W.K. and Rioux, F. (1974), *Pharmacol. Rev.,* **26**, 69–123.

Reid, I.A. (1977), *Circul. Res.,* **41**, 147–153.

Reid, I.A. and Day, R.P. (1977), in: *Central Actions of Angiotensin and Related Hormones.* (Buckley, J.P. and Ferrario, C., eds), Pergamon Press, New York, pp. 267–282.

Renaud, L.P. (1977), in: *Approaches to the Cell Biology of Neurons.* (Cowan, W.M. and Ferrendelli, J.A., eds), Society for Neuroscience, Bethesda, Maryland, pp. 265–290.

Renaud, L.P. and Martin, J.B. (1975), *Brain Res.,* **86**, 150–154.

Renaud, L.P., Martin, J.B. and Brazeau, P. (1975), *Nature,* **255**, 233–235.

Renaud, L.P., Martin, J.B. and Brazeau, P. (1976), *Pharmac. Biochem. Behav.,* **5**, (Suppl. 1), 171–178.

Renaud, L. and Padjen, A. (1978), in: *Centrally Acting Peptides.* (Hughes, J., ed), University Park Press, Baltimore, pp. 59–84.

Renaud, L.P., Pittman, Q.J., Blume, H.W., Lamour, Y. and Arnauld, E. (1979), in: *Central Nervous System Effects of Hypothalamic Hormones and Other Peptides.* (Collu, R., Barbeau, A., Ducharme, J.R. and Rochefort, J.G., eds), Raven Press, New York, pp. 147–161.

Rivier, J.E., Brown, M.R. and Vale, M.W. (1976), *J. med. Chem.,* **19**, 1010–1013.

Rivier, C., Brown, M. and Vale, W. (1977), *Endocrinology,* **100**, 751–754.

Rivier, C., Rivier, J. and Vale, W. (1978), *Endocrinology,* **102**, 519–522.

Robberecht, P., De Neef, P., Lammens, M., Deschodt-Lanckman, M. and Christophe, J.P. (1978), *Eur. J. Biochem.,* **90**, 147–154.

Said, S.I. (1975), in: *Gastrointestinal Hormones.* (Thompson, J.S., ed), University of Texas, Austin, pp. 591–597.

Said, S.I. (1978), in: *Gut Hormones.* (Bloom, S.R., ed), Churchill Livingstone, Edinburgh, pp. 465–469.

Said, S.I. and Mutt, V. (1970), *Science,* **169**, 1217–1218.

Said, S.I. and Mutt, V. (1972), *Eur. J. Biochem.,* **28**, 199–204.

Said, S.I. and Porter, J.C. (1979), *Life Sci.,* **24**, 227–230.

Said, S.I. and Rosenberg, R. (1976), *Science,* **192**, 907–908.

Sakai, K.K., Marks, B.H., George, J. and Koestner, A. (1974), *Life Sci.,* **14**, 1337–1344.

Schaeffer, J.M., Brownstein, M.J. and Axelrod, J. (1977), *Proc. natn. Acad. Sci. USA*, **74**, 3579–3581.

Schally, A.V. (1978), *Science*, **202**, 18–28.

Schonbrunn, A. and Tashjian, A.H. Jr (1978), *J. biol. Chem.*, **253**, 2473–6483.

Severs, W.B. and Daniels-Severs, A.E. (1973), *Pharmacol. Rev.*, **25**, 415–449.

Shiu, R.P.C. and Friesen, H.G. (1974), *Biochem. J.*, **140**, 301–311.

Simpson, J.B., Mangiapane, M.L. and Dellman, H.D. (1978), *Fed. Proc.*, **37**, 2676–2682.

Sirett, N.E., McLean, A.S., Bray, J.J. and Hubbard, J.I. (1977), *Brain Res.*, **122**, 299–312.

Sirett, N.E., Thornton, S.N. and Hubbard, J.I. (1979), *Brain Res.*, **166**, 139–148.

Snyder, S.H. (1978a), in: *Neurobiology of Peptides, Neurosci. Res. Prog. Bull.*, Vol. 16(2). (Iversen, L.L., Nicoll, R.A. and Vale, W.W., eds), MIT Press, Cambridge, Massachusetts, pp. 262–272.

Snyder, S.H. (1978b), in: *The Hypothalamus.* (Reichlin, S., Baldessarini, R.J. and Martin, J.B., eds), Raven Press, New York, pp. 233–243.

Soloff, M., Swartz, T., Morrison, M. and Saffran, M. (1973), *Endocrinology*, **92**, 104–107.

Spiess, J. and Vale, W. (1978), *Metabolism*, **27** (Suppl. 1), 1175–1178.

Stamler, J.F., Raizada, M.K., Phillips, M.I. and Fellows, R.E. (1978), *Physiologist*, **21**(4), 115.

Stanton, T.L., Winokur, A. and Beckman, A.L. (1978), *Neuroscience Abs.*, **4**, 415 (Abs. No. 1314).

Starke, K., Taube, H.D. and Borowski, E. (1977), *Biochem. Pharmacol.*, **26**, 259–268.

Swanson, L.W. (1978), *Neuroscience Abs.*, **4**, 415 (Abs. No. 1316).

Swanson, L.W., Marshall, G.R., Needleman, P. and Sharpe, L.G. (1973), *Brain Res.*, **49**, 441–446.

Tan, A.T., Tsang, D., Renaud, L.P. and Martin, J.B. (1977), *Brain Res.*, **123**, 193–196.

Taraskevich, P.S. and Douglas, W.W. (1977), *Proc. natn. Acad. Sci. USA*, **74**, 4064–4067.

Tashjian, A.H., Barowsky, N.J. and Hensen, D.K. (1971), *Biochem. biophys. Res. Commun.*, **43**, 516–523.

Taylor, D.P. and Pert, C.B. (1979), *Proc. natn. Acad. Sci. USA*, **76**, 660–664.

Taylor, R.L. and Burt, D.R. (1980), *Proc. endocrine Soc.*, 62nd Meet., in press (Abstract).

Terry, L.C. and Martin, J.B. (1978), *Ann. Rev. Pharmacol. Toxicol.*, **18**, 111–123.

Tixier-Vidal, A., Gourdji, D., Pradelles, P., Morgat, J.L., Fromageot, P. and Kerdelhué, B. (1975), in: *Hypothalamic Hormones*, (Motta, M., Crosignani, P.G. and Martini, L., eds), Academic Press, New York, pp. 89–107.

Uhl, G.R., Bennett, J.P. Jr and Snyder, S.H. (1977a), *Brain Res.*, **130**, 299–313.

Uhl, G.R., Goodman, R.R. and Snyder, S.H. (1979), *Brain Res.*, **167**, 77–91.

Uhl, G.R., Kuhar, M.J. and Snyder, S.H. (1977b), *Proc. natn. Acad. Sci. USA*, **74**, 4059–4063.

Uhl, G.R. and Snyder, S.H. (1976), *Life Sci.*, **19**, 1827–1832.

Uhl, G.R. and Snyder, S.H. (1977), *Eur. J. Pharmacol.*, **41**, 89–91.

Vale, W., Grant, G. and Guillemin, R. (1973), in: *Frontiers in Neuroendocrinology.* (Ganong, W.F. and Martini, L., eds), Oxford University Press, London, pp. 375–413.

Vale, W., Rivier, C. and Brown, M. (1977), *Ann. Rev. Physiol.,* **39**, 473–527.

Vale, W., Rivier, J. and Burgus, R. (1971), *Endocrinology,* **89**, 1485–1488.

Vale, W., Rivier, J., Ling, N. and Brown, M. (1978), *Metabolism,* **27** (Suppl. 1), 1391–1401.

Veber, D.F., Holly, F.W., Varga, S.L., Hirschmann, R., Nutt, R.F., Lotti, V.J. and Porter, C.C. (1977), *Peptides 1976: Proceedings of the Fourteenth European Peptide Symposium,* (Loffett, A., ed), University of Brussels Press, Brussels, Belgium, pp. 453–461.

Vijayan, E., Samson, W.K., Said, S.I. and McCann, S.M. (1979), *Endocrinology,* **104**, 53–57.

Villarreal, J.A. and Brown, M.R. (1978), *Life Sci.,* **23**, 2729–2734.

Wei, E., Loh, H. and Way, E.L. (1976), *Eur. J. Pharmacol.,* **36**, 227–229.

Wharton, J., Polak, J.M., Bloom, S.R., Ghate, M.A., Solcia, E., Brown, M.R. and Pearse, A.G.E. (1978), *Nature,* **273**, 769–770.

Whittaker, V.P., Michaelson, I.A. and Kirkland, R.J.A. (1964), *Biochem. J.,* **90**, 293–303.

Wilber, J.F., Montoya, E., Plotnikoff, N.P., White, W.F., Gendrich, R., Renaud, L. and Martin, J.B. (1976), *Rec. Prog. Hormone Res.,* **32**, 117–159.

Winokur, A. and Utiger, R.D. (1974), *Science,* **185**, 265–267.

Winokur, A. and Utiger, R.D. (1979), in: *Central Nervous Actions of Hypothalamic Hormones and Other Peptides.* (Collu, R., Barbeau, A., Ducharme, J.R. and Rochefort, J.G., eds), Raven Press, New York, pp. 55–63.

Yarbrough, G.G. (1976), *Nature,* **263**, 523–524.

Young, W., Uhl, G. and Kuhar, M. (1978), *Brain Res.,* **150**, 431–435.

Youngblood, W.W., Humm, J. and Kizer, J.S. (1979), *Brain Res.,* **163**, 101–110.

Youngblood, W.W., Lipton, M.A. and Kizer, J.S. (1978), *Brain Res.,* **151**, 99–116.

Index

References to figures and tables are in italics.